Practical
Physical Pharmacy

(As Per B.Pharm Syllabus of Various Universities & Education Governing Bodies)

W0193084

Practical
Physical Pharmacy

(As Per B.Pharm Syllabus of Various Universities & Education Governing Bodies)

Prof. R.S. GAUD

M.Pharm. , Ph.D. , F.I.C.

Dr. G.D. GUPTA

M.Pharm. , Ph.D.
Assistant Professor,
L.M. College of Science & Technology (Pharmacy)
Jodhpur

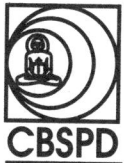

CBSPD

CBS Publishers & Distributors Pvt Ltd

New Delhi • Bengaluru • Chennai • Kochi • Kolkata • Lucknow • Mumbai
Hyderabad • Jharkhand • Nagpur • Patna • Pune • Uttarakhand

Practical Physical Pharmacy

ISBN: 978-81-239-0737-6

First Edition: 2001

Reprint: 2003, 2005, 2006, 2007, 2008, 2009, 2010, 2012, 2016, 2019, 2020, 2023

Published by Satish Kumar Jain and produced by Varun Jain for

CBS Publishers & Distributors Pvt Ltd
4819/XI Prahlad Street, 24 Ansari Road, Daryaganj, New Delhi 110 002, India
Ph: 011-23289259, 23266861   Website: www.cbspd.com
                                   e-mail: delhi@cbspd.com
Corporate Office: 204 FIE, Industrial Area, Patparganj, Delhi 110 092
Ph: 011-4934 4934   Fax: 011-4934 4935   e-mail: publishing@cbspd.com
                                               publicity@cbspd.com

Branches

- **Bengaluru:** Seema House 2975, 17th Cross, KR Road, Banasankari 2nd Stage, Bengaluru 560 070, Karnataka, India
  Ph: +91-80-26771678/79   Fax: +91-80-26771680   e-mail: bangalore@cbspd.com
- **Chennai:** 7, Subbaraya Street, Shenoy Nagar, Chennai 600 030, Tamil Nadu, India
  Ph: +91-44-26680620, 26681266   Fax: +91-44-42032115   e-mail: chennai@cbspd.com
- **Kochi:** 42/1325, 1326, Power House Road, Opp KSEB, Power House, Ernakulam 682 018, India
  Ph: +91-484-4059061-65   Fax: +91-484-4059065   e-mail: kochi@cbspd.com
- **Kolkata:** 147, Hind Ceramics Compound, 1st Floor, Nilgunj Road, Belghoria, Kolkata 700 056, West Bengal, India
  Ph: +91-9096713055/56   e-mail: kolkata@cbspd.com
- **Lucknow:** Basement, Khushnuma Complex, 7-Meerabai Marg (behind Jawahar Bhawan), Lucknow 226 001, India
  Ph: +91-522-4000032   e-mail: tiwari.lucknow@cbspd.com
- **Mumbai:** PWD Shed. Gala no. 25/26, Ramchandra Bhatt Marg, Next to JJ Hospital Gate no. 2, Opp. Union Bank of India
  Noorbaug Mumbai 400 009, Maharashtra, India
  Ph: +91-22-66661880/89   e-mail: mumbai@cbspd.com

Representatives

• **Hyderabad**	0-9885175004	• **Jharkhand**	0-9811541605	• **Nagpur**	0-9421945513
• **Patna**	0-9334159340	• **Pune**	0-9923910676	• **Uttarakhand**	0-9716462459

Printed at Neekunj Print Process, Haryana

Preface

Physical pharmacy comprises mainly of principles of basic sciences as these are applied in pharmacy and allied industries. The subject has been taught ever since the very inception of pharmacy education though initially it was introduced as a part of general pharmacy.

Due to its important role in creating an understanding of the basic principles involved in pharmacy practice, it evolved as a separate course over time. Adequate emphasis, befitting its foundation-laying nature, began to be given to its teaching and consequently to fulfil the market need many books have also been written on this topic. Unfortunately, most of the books have considered only the theoretical aspect of this subject. The Authors, considering this lacuna, have attempted to fulfil this gap.

The book has been divided into thirteen chapters based on the priority areas of the subject covering model syllabus of AICTE. The principles involved, the required theoretical background, procedures involved, precautions to be taken in the laboratory and the question bank for viva voce have all been discussed at large.

Authors have tried to frame up good number of exercises covering all important subject matters, which a pharmacy student must perform in the laboratory.

We sincerely hope the book will be useful to all students of pharmacy and allied sciences in understanding the basic principles involved in pharma practices.

Authors are thankful to Mr. H. S. Poplai, General Manager, M/s CBS Publishers & Distributors and his team for their sincere efforts in publishing this book in the present form.

Constructive suggestions, if any, will be appreciated.

Prof. R.S. Gaud
Dr. G.D. Gupta

ABOUT THE BOOK

It was suggested by many of the teachers engaged in the field of pharmacy that there is a need for practical manual of physical pharmacy as it is the foundation course for pharmaceutics. Authors took this task upon themselves resulting in publication of this book entitled "Practical Physical Pharmacy".

The book comprises of ninety-one exercises in thirteen chapters. Each exercise is presented covering basic principles, theoretical background, material requirements, procedures, observations, calculations and precautions to be taken in the laboratory and question bank at the end of each exercise for viva voce.

Chapter One, Introduction deals with importance of Physical Pharmacy and the laboratory behavior viz. Handling and cleaning of glassware, laboratory safety, laboratory manners and the way to write exercise in journal, common errors and their solution with suitable examples considered in this chapter.

Other chapters viz. Molecular Weight, Density of liquids, Rheology, Surface tension, Solubility, Vapor pressure, Partition coefficient, Phase rule, Colloids, Refractivity, Chemical kinetics and Micromeritics include the various exercises related to the basis of physicochemical characteristics of substances, method of determination, factor affecting the methods viz. temperature, pressure, addition of impurities and other parameters with suitable models using simple as well as effective techniques to get reproducible results. Mathematical approach involved for justification of various problems has been discussed wherever necessary.

Sincere efforts have been made to make it an ideal practical book on Physical Pharmacy and the book is also useful for science graduates studying physical chemistry. The book is presented in simple language with illustrative diagrams, flow charts and graphs as per the need of the syllabus.

ABOUT THE AUTHORS

Dr. G.D. Gupta, M.Pharm, Ph.D., is Assistant Professor in Pharmaceutics at L.M. College of Science & Technology, Jodhpur, Rajasthan since last five years. He has published and presented many research papers at national and international journals/conferences.

Dr. Gupta has delivered many guest lectures and participated as a resource person in workshops sponsored by AICTE and UGC. Recently he has been awarded 'Best Paper Award' in 5th APTI National Convention. Dr.Gupta has also authored three professional books.

He is a life member of pharmaceutical societies and is actively involved in professional organizations.

Prof. R.S.Gaud, M.Pharm, Ph.D., is a professor of pharmaceutics and engaged in teaching and research since 1978 in the Dept. of Pharmacy, Indore, Madhya Pradesh. Currently he is working with All India Council for Technical Education, New Delhi, an autonomous body under the Govt. of India Parliament Act, 1987 as Advisor.

He started his career as lecturer in Pharmacy, Holkar Science College, Indore and served in various capacities in the institutions viz. Asst. Professor and Professor in S.G.S. Institute of Science & Technology, Indore and Principal, AISSMS College of Pharmacy, Pune.

He was also Dean, Faculty of Technology, and Member, Executive Council, Devi Ahilya Vishwavidyalaya, Indore. He is also actively involved in many academic organizations at national and international levels.

He has established himself as a good teacher and researcher and has participated and presented many research papers at national and international levels. He has visited Bangkok (Thailand), Amsterdam (Holland), Vancouver (Canada), Chicago, Madison, New Orleans (USA). He is the author of many books, research papers and review articles in the field of pharmaceutics.

Prof. Gaud has rendered his valuable services to most of the universities in the country for their academic upliftment. He is a life member of various pharmaceutical societies and was Vice-President, Association of Pharmacy Teachers in India.

Contents

PREFACE   **V**

Chapter 1.   **INTRODUCTION**   **1-11**

Handling of Glasswares   2

Laboratory Safety   3

Avoid in Laboratory   4

Laboratory Manners   5

How to Write Exercise   6

Chapter 2.   **MOLECULAR WEIGHT**   **12-28**

EXERCISE NO. 2.1   14

To determine molecular weight of volatile substance by Victor Meyer's Method

EXERCISE NO. 2.2   16

To estimate composition of a binary mixture of volatile liquids by Vector Meyer's method

EXERCISE NO. 2.3   19

To determine molecular weight of liquid by steam distillation method

EXERCISE NO. 2.4   21

To determine molecular weight of non-volatile substance using water as solvent.

EXERCISE NO. 2.5   23

To determine molecular weight of a non-electrolyte substance using benzene as solvent

EXERCISE NO. 2.6   24

To determine molecular weight of a given substance by Landsberger mehtod

EXERCISE NO. 2.7

To determine molecular weight of a substance by Rast-Camphor method   26

Viva-voce Question Bank   28

Chapter 3.   **DENSITY OF LIQUIDS**   **29-45**

EXERCISE NO. 3.1   33

Determine Density of Water at different Temperature using Pycnometer

EXERCISE NO. 3.2   35

Determine density of given liquid at a definite temperature using (a) Density bottle (b) Pycnometer

EXERCISE NO. 3.3   37
To study the effect of temperature on density of given
liquid using Pycnometer.
EXERCISE NO. 3.4   38
To study the effect of temperature on density of given
liquid using density bottle.
EXERCISE NO. 3.5   39
To study the effect of salt viz. sodium chloride in different
concentration on the density of water at 25°C or room
temperature.
EXERCISE NO. 3.6   41
To prepare different concentration of sucrose in purified
waters and determine density at room temperature using
density bottle and pycnometer.
EXERCISE NO. 3.7   42
To prepare different composition of glycerine and water
and determine density at room temperature.(for accuracy
provide unknown samples).
EXERCISE NO. 3.8   43
Determine the molal volume of ethanol at 25°C or room
temperature.
Viva-voce Question Bank   45

Chapter 4.   **RHEOLOGY**   **46-80**
Determination of Viscosity   50
EXERCISE NO. 4.1   55
To determine viscosity of liquid using Ostwald's
viscometer at room temperature
EXERCISE NO. 4.2   57
To determine viscosity of liquid using Falling ball
viscometer
EXERCISE NO. 4.3   60
To determine viscosity of liquid using Redwood
viscometer
EXERCISE NO. 4.4   63
To determine viscosity of paracetamol suspension/
shampoo using Ostwald's viscometer
EXERCISE NO. 4.5   65
To determine viscosity of calamine lotion using Redwood
viscometer
EXERCISE NO. 4.6   66
To determine viscosity of liquid paraffin emulsion using
Falling ball viscometer

EXERCISE NO. 4.7   67
To determine viscosity of Shampoo using Ostwald's
viscometer
EXERCISE NO. 4.8   68
To study the effect of temperature on viscosity
EXERCISE NO. 4.9   70
To study the effect of concentration on viscosity
EXERCISE NO. 4.10   72
To prepare different composition of glycerin and water and
determine viscosity using Ostwald's viscometer
EXERCISE NO. 4.11   74
To determine composition of liquids by viscosity
EXERCISE NO. 4.12   75
To determine viscosity of gel using Brookfield viscometer
EXERCISE NO. 4.13   77
To determine viscosity of simple ointment using
Brookfield viscometer
EXERCISE NO. 4.14   78
To study the effect of impurities on viscosity
EXERCISE NO. 4.15   79
To study the effect of polarity on viscosity (ethanol,glycol
and glycerol)
Viva-voce Question Bank   80

Chapter 5.   SURFACE TENSION   81-105
Classification of Interfaces   81
Surface tension   ·81
Surface Free Energy   83
Methods for Measurement of surface tension and   84
interfacial tension
EXERCISE NO. 5.1   87
To determine surface tension of liquid using
stalagmometer.
EXERCISE NO. 5.2   89
To determine surface tension of liquid using capillary rise
method.
EXERCISE NO. 5.3   91
To determine surface tension of liquid using DuNouy
tensiometer.
EXERCISE NO. 5.4   93
To determine parachor of given liquid by surface tension
method using stalagmometer

EXERCISE NO. 5.5   95
To determine surface tension of benzene and n-hexane
using stalagmometer.
EXERCISE NO. 5.6   97
To study the effect of temperature on surface tension.
EXERCISE NO. 5.7   98
To study the effect of concentration on surface tension.
EXERCISE NO. 5.8   100
To prepare different composition of glycerin and water and
determine surface tension using stalagmometer.
EXERCISE NO. 5.9   101
To determine composition of liquids by surface tension.
EXERCISE NO. 5.10   102
To study the effect of surfactant on surface tension.
EXERCISE NO. 5.11   103
To study the effect of impurities on surface tension.
EXERCISE NO. 5.12   104
To study the effect of polarity on surface tension.(ethanol
and glycol).
Viva-voce Question Bank   105

Chapter 6.   **SOLUBILITY**   **106-125**
Solubility   106
Expression of Solubility   107
Factors Affecting Solubility   107
Determination of Solubility   108
EXERCISE NO. 6.1   110
To determine the solubility of an inorganic salt at different
temperature.
EXERCISE NO. 6.2   112
To determine the solubility of benzoic acid at room
temperature and below the room temperature (10°C) by
volumetric method.
EXERCISE NO. 6.3   115
To determine the heat of solution of substance by solubility
method
EXERCISE NO. 6.4   116
To study the effect of additive of an electrolyte on the
solubility of an organic acid at room temperature
EXERCISE NO. 6.5   118
To study the effect of temperature on solubility of
paracetamol

EXERCISE NO. 6.6   120
To study the effect of stirring on solubility of paracetamol
EXERCISE NO. 6.7   121
To study the effect of particle size on solubility
EXERCISE NO. 6.8   123
To study the effect of solubilizing agent on solubilization
Viva-voce Question Bank   125

Chapter 7.   VAPOR PRESSURE   126-138
Factors Affecting Vapor Pressure   127
Determination of Vapor Pressure   128
EXERCISE NO. 7.1   130
To determine vapor pressure of pure water at different
temperature
EXERCISE NO. 7.2   132
To determine the vapor pressure of benzene at different
temperature
EXERCISE NO. 7.3   134
To determine the vapor pressure of benzene at different
temperature using Ramsay-Young apparatus
EXERCISE NO. 7.4   136
To determine the vapor pressure of carbon tetrachloride
using as isoteniscope.
Viva-voce Question Bank   138

Chapter 8.   PARTITION COEFFICIENT   139-151
EXERCISE NO. 8.1   142
To determine the partition coefficient of iodine between
carbon tetrachloride and distilled water
EXERCISE NO. 8.2   145
To determine the partition coefficient of succinic acid
between ether and distilled water
EXERCISE NO. 8.3   147
To determine the partition coefficient of succinic acid
between benzene and distilled water
EXERCISE NO. 8.4   148
To determine the partition coefficient of benzoic acid in
benzene and distilled water
Viva-voce Question Bank   151

Chapter 9.   PHASE RULE   152-160
EXERCISE NO. 9.1   154
To determine critical solution temperature of phenol and
water

EXERCISE NO. 9.2   156
To study the effect of substances on the solubility of two
immiscible liquids
EXERCISE NO. 9.3   158
To determine the composition and the amounts of layer
obtained by mixing phenol and distilled water in equal
proportion
EXERCISE NO. 9.4   159
To study a solubility curve of a ternary system
Viva-voce Question Bank   160

Chapter 10.   **COLLOIDS**   **161-183**
Characteristics of Colloids   161
Classification of Colloids   162
Method of Preparation   163
Properties of Colloids   163
Some Important Terminology   165
EXERCISE NO. 10.1   167
To prepare and study colloidal solution of arsenic sulphide
EXERCISE NO. 10.2   169
To prepare and study colloidal solution of ferric hydroxide
EXERCISE NO. 10.3   170
To prepare and study colloidal solution of silver
EXERCISE NO. 10.4   171
To prepare and study colloidal solution of gelatin
EXERCISE NO. 10.5   172
To study the effect of sodium chloride, (monovalent),
barium chloride (divalent), and aluminium chloride
(trivalent) on arsenic sulphate sol
EXERCISE NO. 10.6   175
To determine the effect of potassium chloride and
potassium sulphate on ferric hydroxide sols
EXERCISE NO. 10.7   176
To study the protective action of hydrophilic colloid on the
precipitation of a hydrophobic colloids
EXERCISE NO. 10.8   178
To determine the optimum ratio for precipitation
EXERCISE NO. 10.9   180
To determine the charge on the particles in a given
colloidal solution and determine zeta potential
Viva-voce Question Bank   182

Chapter 11.   **REFRACTIVITY**   **184-191**
Snell's Law of Refraction   184
Measurement of Refractive Index   185
EXERCISE NO. 11.1   186
To determine refractive index of a given liquid using Abbe
refractometer
EXERCISE NO. 11.2   188
To study the effect of temperature on refractive index by
Abbe refrectometer
EXERCISE NO. 11.3   190
To determine the effect of concentration on refrective
index by Abbe refrectometer
Viva-voce Question Bank   191

Chapter 12.   **CHEMICAL KINETICS**   **192-205**
Rate of reaction   192
Factor Influencing Rate of Reaction   193
Order of Reaction   193
Determination of Order of Reaction   195
EXERCISE NO. 12.1   196
To determine velocity constant of the hydrolysis of given
compound
EXERCISE NO. 12.2   198
To determine the relative strength of two acids
EXERCISE NO. 12.3   200
To determine the saponification value of given ester
EXERCISE NO. 12.4   203
To investigate the reaction between acetone and iodine
Viva-voce Question Bank   205

Chapter 13.   **MICROMERITICS**   **206-230**
Particle Size and Size Distribution   207
Characterization of Powder Size   208
Determination of Particle Size   209
EXERCISE NO. 13.1   211
To determine the particle size of powder by sieving
method
EXERCISE NO. 13.2   213
To determine particle of size in disperse medium by
microscopic method
EXERCISE NO. 13.3   215
To determine globule size of emulsion by microscopic
method

EXERCISE NO. 13.4   216
To determine particle of size disperse medium by sedimentation method
EXERCISE NO. 13.5   218
To determine surface area of the particles by permeability method
EXERCISE NO. 13.6   219
To determine the true density of given powder by solvent displacement method
EXERCISE NO. 13.7   220
To determine the true density of given powder by compressed power method
EXERCISE NO. 13.8   221
To determine the bulk density of the given powder
EXERCISE NO. 13.9   222
To determine the granule density of given sample
EXERCISE NO. 13.10   223
To determine porosity, intra-particle porosity, interspace or void porosity and total porosity of powder
EXERCISE NO. 13.11   224
To determine the angle of repose of the given powder material
EXERCISE NO. 13.12   225
To study the effect of glidant on flow properties of powder
EXERCISE NO. 13.13   226
To determine compressibility index of powder
EXERCISE NO. 13.14   228
To determine dispersibility of powder using hollow cylindrical method
Viva-voce Question Bank   229

Appendix   **231-238**
Table 1. Some commonly used physicochemical costants   231
Table 2. Symbols and Abbrebiation   232
Table 3. Greek Alphabets   232
Table 4. Physical Quantities   233
Table 5. Atomic number and atomic mass of elements   233
Table 6. Surface tension of liquids at 20°C   236
Table 7. Interfacial tension of liquids against water at 20°C   236
Table 8. Physical constant of water at different temperature   237
Table 9. Appropriate viscosity of liquids   238

Chapter 1

INTRODUCTION

Physical pharmacy is a backbone of the pharmacy. It covers many principles and mathematical models, related not only to formulation of dosage forms but also to all those principles related to synthesis of the compounds. It is an intermediate subject between chemistry and pharmaceutics and covers many topics like stability of products, kinetics of drug release, effect of heat on drug, ionization, acid and base balance. While practicing pharmacy one has to depend on principles involved in basic science. Pharmacist utilizes principles and methods derived from other branches of science.

Modernization has created a stress in the minds of professionals and every body has to demonstrate the proper application of knowledge gained from other sources. Thus all those basic principles of science used in the practice of pharmacy are grouped together and studied under the physical pharmacy.

Physical pharmacy being an applied science, the physical and quantitative principles involved in implementing duties as a chemist or formulation chemist or pharmacologist are derived from basic science and success of pharmacist mainly depends on his capability of utilizing his knowledge based on such principles.

For rapid development of profession pharmacist has to update his knowledge in the field of physical pharmacy. The principles involved are simple to understand in the modern era of information technology and drug delivery system. In the modern era most of the instruments are attached with computer.

Physical pharmacy includes the basic knowledge of all those pharmacist who are working in field viz. industries, teaching, manufacturing, retail pharmacy, marketing and any of the allied branches of the profession. In all fields sound knowledge of physical pharmacy with computer application is essential to handle the instruments and application in the mathematical operations. Physical pharmacy has been related to the many field of the pharmacy profession viz.

- Analytical chemistry
- Medicinal chemistry
- Formulation of dosage forms
- Stability studies
- Pharmacokinetics and biopharmaceutics
- Pharmacology
- Pharmacognosy
- Biochemistry
- Organic chemistry
- Medicinal chemistry
- Synthesis of drugs
- Computer application in pharmacy

HANDING OF GLASSWARES

Laboratory glassware are usually manufactured from borosilicate glass. The heat, reagents, solvents or any chemicals do not affect it. Borosilicate mainly contains silica, boric acid, sodium oxide and aluminium oxide.

Washing of glasswares

1. After using the glassware, wash the glassware with the running tap water immediately.
2. Use scrubber and detergent to clean the glassware and wash with water.
3. Further rinse the glassware thoroughly with tap water.
4. Tissue culture glassware should be washed with the 5% detergent solution for three to four times.
5. The automatic washer is used only as a rinsing unit and no detergent is to be added in the washing process. Glassware should be treated with detergent prior to its transfer into the washing system.
6. The automatic washer is programmed for not less than six washings with tap water and then rinse with distilled water for about 1 min.
7. If automatic washer is not provided then wash manually at least four times with the tap water.
8. Soak new glassware for some time in 1% hydrochloric acid solution since new glassware is slightly alkaline in reaction, which may affect the results.
9. If glassware has been contaminated with the media or any other types of contamination that is very difficult to remove prior treatment with the nitric acid, or chromic acid reagent is required.

Drying of Glasswares

After washing and draining excess water, glassware are to be dried. Volumetric type of glassware should be dried in the hot air oven. Common glassware can be dried at room temperature. It can be dried by rubbing with dry cloth or towel. Dried glassware should be protected from dust and other types of contamination. If necessary cover them with cloth or wrap in brown-paper. For instant drying, hair-drier can also be utilized.

Heating and cooling of glasswares

1. Never leave the containers unattended when you are heating the container. Sometimes some serious problem may arise as over heating at high temperature may result in cracking the glassware or accident may take place.
2. Do not put hot glassware on a damp surface.
3. Cool the glassware slowly to prevent thermal breakage.
4. Heat all liquids slowly and always use metallic-wire gauze or water bath to diffuse heat.

Precautions

1. Re-usable glassware should be emptied immediately after use.
2. Never leave sticky material in the glasswares.
3. Segregate all those glassware that contain corrosive chemicals.
4. Contaminated Glassware should be decontaminated before washing.
5. Remove the label before washing the glassware.
6. Rubber lined screw caps should be soaked only in distilled water. Never soak caps in detergent or soap solution.
7. Glassware should be rinsed with the same solvent or solution to be used with the glassware, before taking in use.
8. Put proper label on the glassware. In case of any confusion do not take risks without conforming or discard it.

LABORATORY SAFETY

In the laboratory, safety is necessary because many sensitive, poisonous and dangerous substances and microorganisms surround it. Several precautions are required to be taken such as

- Handling of broken glasswares
- Handling of injurious substances
- Inhalation of poisonous fumes or gases
- Handling of corrosive reagents
- Handling of substances in aseptic room

- Cleaning of glasswares
- Handling of machinery and equipments
- Handling of electric points
- Handling of inflammable substances

LABORATORY FIRST AID

Laboratory first aid kit should contain following materials

- Absorbent cotton wool and gauze
- Bandage
- Disposable syringe
- Medicated adhesive tape
- Diluted ethyl alcohol
- Iodine tincture
- A disinfectant solution
- Forceps (Two)
- Scissors (Two)
- Sterilized saline solution
- Soap solution
- Common medicines such as

    i. Anti-emetics
    ii. Antacid preparations
    iii. Analgesics/Antipyretic
    iv. Antibiotic preparation
    v. Paracetamol tablets
    vi. Antihistaminic formulations
    vii. Eye wash
    viii. Eye ointment
    ix. Soframycin ointment

AVOID IN LABORATORY

1. Hand shaking
2. Drinking or eating
3. Laughing
4. Sneezing without covering the mouth
5. Cutting nails with teeth
6. Smoking
7. Sucking corrosive solutions using pipette
8. Spitting in the laboratory

9. Touching corrosive/hazardous substances
10. Group discussion (unnecessary taking)
11. Transferring of fire using papers
12. Opening bottle by mouth
13. Using duster for cleaning body surfaces
14. Using hanky for holding glasswarees

LABORATORY MANNERS

1. Do not enter in the laboratory without wearing apron and essential requirement in the laboratory.
2. Clean your working space and keep things limited to requirement of your current exercise.
3. Do not borrow or lend anything to your colleague.
4. Do not light your burner with adjacent burner or transfer fire by means.
5. Keep your burner off when it is not in use.
6. Do not blow off the burner by mouth.
7. Keep your journal in safe area away from wash basin or working bench. Preferably cover it with waterproof material.
8. Do not discuss anything with your colleague or a group during practical. Contact your teacher if you have queries.
9. Always use dustbin for throwing waste material and do not use wash basin for this act.
10. Do not clean culture or smear plates in the wash basin. Treat it with disinfectant and then clean it.
11. Always sterilize inoculating loop or needle by holding it vertically on the flame before and after its use.
12. Gas leakage, if any should be immediately reported to your lab technician or teacher.
13. If you have any injury during practical, leave the laboratory and contact your office or teacher for first aid box.
14. Do not go outside with your apron and without washing your hands with detergent and disinfectant.
15. Do not carry costly things likely to be lost in the laboratory.
16. Preferably do not use cosmetics in the laboratory.
17. While leaving the laboratory, clean your working table with disinfectant.
18. Check water and gas connections before leaving the laboratory.
19. Leave the laboratory and use preparation room to remove your apron, mask and hair cover. Fold and pack it in a separate plastic cover and keep it for fumigation.
20. Clean your hand with soap and then with disinfectant. Finally, rewash it with fresh water.

BESIDE THE MAIN CODE OF CONDUCT AND DISCIPLINE IN THE LABORATORY

Things to be checked before entering in laboratory

1. Record file with cover
2. Small note book
3. Neat and clean apron
4. Compass box, black and colored pencils, scale, sharpener, eraser and compass tools
5. Match box/lighter
6. Needle
7. Glass marker
8. Ready made glued labels of different size
9. White sheet for working table
10. Neat and clean napkin
11. Fractional weight box
12. Other necessary materials as per the requirement of the experiments

Check whether you know?

1. Object of the experiment
2. Requirement of the exercise
3. Purpose or application of experiment
4. Methodology adopted
5. Principle involved
6. Instruments to be used
7. Operation or handling of instruments and equipments
8. Outcome expected
9. Precautions
10. Where you stand in above respect

How to Write Exercise?

Journal size should be minimum of 250 pages for 30 exercises in a session. Occasionally, specific record is provided by the institute. In that case use as per the instructions given by your teacher.

Journal should be covered with waterproof paper. Do not use colored or fluorescent paper, newspaper, magazine paper etc. for cover.

Prepare a label with following information and fix it properly in the center/left corner of cover page of the record and inside the record-book. e.g.

Name	Roll No.
Session	Subject
Name of Institute	

Open your record book, leave first page for certificate to be given by the institute for completion of record at the end of the session. Leave second and third page blank. This gives few moments to think about you to the observer and create a good impression.

Make index having at least four page which covers following informations

S. No.	Experiment No.	Object	Date	Page No.	Marks / Grade	Signature / Remarks

Start your experiment with fresh page, Journal contains two types of pages, blank on left hand side and ruled on right hand side. Use these sides as mentioned in the following columns.

Blank page information	Ruled page information
• Requirements • Formula or Table if any • Observation (tabular form if required) • Flow diagram of working procedure • Diagram of special equipment you have used for the experiment • Conclusion • Result*	• Date • Exercise No. • Serial No. • Page No. • Object • Theory • Procedure • Result • Applications • Precautions • References

On the first page

Date	Experiment No.	Page No.

• Object
• References
• Theory

	Do's	Don't
1. Date	July 15, 2000	J-15, 2000
	or 10.01.2000	J-15, 00
	or 10.01.2000	15th July –00
	or 10.01.2 K	15.01.00
2. Experiment No.	Experiment No.	Ex. NO.
	EXPERIMENT No.	ep. no.
3. Page No.	2	Two
		II
	02	2nd
4. Serial Number	S. No.	Serial NO.
	Serial No.	S.no.
5. Object	Object :	OBJECT :
	Object :-	ObJect:
	OBJECT :	ObjecT :

REFERENCES

Though there are many sources of information but in the laboratory there are only three types of sources of information.

(a) Reference book

(b) Textbook or hand book

(c) Journals

Following rule is generally followed by many for writing the references in the laboratory journals.

(a) Last name, initials, name of the other writers in the same way, name of the text book, year, edition, publisher, page no.

(b) Last name, initials, name of other writers in the same way, 'name of the reference book' year, edition, publisher, page no.

(c) Last name, initials, name of the other writers in the same way, Name of Journal, year, edition, page no.

---

*Result can be written on either side. Ideal place for the information on ruled side of your record

Theory

In theory one should includes principle, formula, definition, purpose, classification and other related information about the experiments which are helpful to viva voce for theoretical approach. Do not give irrelevant things related to topic, which you are dealing in the experiment.

Procedure

It is always better to use stepwise procedure, the step you have worked in the laboratory and it should be in the past tense as you are narrating the way you have worked for the experiments. Instead of steps, you can write in a regular telegraphic language while writing the procedure. Preferably use minimum sentence or words but it should have sufficient information about the experiment.

Result

At the end of the experiment, you have to judge your observation with the object you have planned before starting the experiment. Summarize the result and give in compact and truthful manner.

How to Face Viva-voce?

No any fixed criterion is there for viva-voce (oral), but it has been observed that the general criterion for distribution of subject matter is as follows :
(a) Related to experiment in the journal   - 20%
(b) Related to the theory of the subject   - 60%
(c) General information   - 10%

Questions Generally Asked

1. What is the aim of your experiment?
2. How to perform this experiment?
3. What is the principle of the experiment?
4. Questions related to techniques.
5. Questions related to aims.
6. Alternative method for the experiment.
7. Reported method of the same.
8. What is the significance of the experiments?
9. Define terminology related to the experiments.
10. Name the equipment and principle of used in the experiments.
11. Miscellaneous questions.

Table 1.1. List of common glasswares & other miscellaneous items

S.N.	Name	S.N.	Name
1.	Beakers 1000,500,250,100,50,ml	21.	Pestle mortars (porcelin, glass)
2.	Burettes 50,100 ml (punch clip, glass stopper)	22.	Pipettes graduated 10,5, 2, 1 ml
		23.	Pipette with bulb 10,20,25,50 ml
3.	Burette clip (steel, teflon, iron)	24.	Petri dishes 4",6"(glass & PVC)
4.	Buchner funnel (porcelin)	25.	Round bottom flask
5.	Conical flask 500,250,100,50, ml (marked, without marked)	26.	R.D.bottle 5,10, 25 ml
		27.	Roux bottle
6.	Conical percolators (steel, glass)	28.	Slides
7.	China dishes	29.	Separating funnel
8.	Clamps (steel, teflon)	30.	Spatula
9.	Centrifuge	31.	Test tubes
10.	Dispensing bottle	32.	Test tube stands
11.	Desiccator (simple or vacuum)	33.	Thermometer(0-110°C,0-360°C)
12.	Erlenmeyer flask	34.	Test tube holders
13.	Funnel 2", 3", 4"(glass & plastic)	35.	Tripod stand
14.	Filtration flask , 500, 250,100 ml	36.	Tubes (open, screw cap, cap)
15.	Flat bottom flask	37.	Volumetric flask 250,100,50, ml
16.	Glass tubes	38.	Weighing bottles
17.	Halfmann clips	39.	Water bath (constant level)
18.	Iodine flasks	40.	Wire gauge
19.	Kolle flasks	41.	Watch glasses
20.	Measuring cylinder	42.	Wash bottles

Table 1.2. List of common equipments

S.No.	Name of Equipment	S.No.	Name of Equipment
1.	Autoclave	25.	Oculometer
2.	Andreasen apparatus	26.	Osmosis apparatus
3.	Brookfield viscometer	27.	Ostwald viscometer
4.	Cup and bob viscometer	28.	Plane slide
5.	Cone and plate viscometer	29	Pipette dryer
6.	Conductivity meter	30.	Plastic carboys
7.	Coulter counter apparatus	31.	Pycnometer
8.	Desiccator cabinet	32.	Polarimeter
9.	Distillation apparatus	33.	Refrigerator
10.	DuNouy tensiometer	34.	Refractometer
11.	Density bottle	35.	Redwood viscometer
12.	Digital pH meter	36.	Separating funnel
13.	Dissolution apparatus	37.	Stalagmometer
14.	Diffusion cell for permeation	38.	Stage micrometer
15.	Electrophoresis	39.	Sieve shaker
16.	Falling sphere viscometer	40.	Sieve set
17.	Glassware Dryer	41	Test tube rotator/ centrifuge
18.	Glass pH electrode	42.	Trays and baskets
19.	Heating mental	43.	UV-chamber
20.	Hot plates	44.	Vapor pressure osmometer
21.	Hot air oven	45.	Vacuum oven
22.	Incubator	46.	Vortex shaker
23.	Metabolic shaker	47.	Water bath
24.	Microscope	48.	Zeta meter

□□□

Chapter 2

MOLECULAR WEIGHT

The molecular weight of a compound is the weight of the molecule of it as compared to the weight of an atom of hydrogen.

Molecular weight = Weight of imperial formula × n

where n = 1, 2, 3, ------ etc., if n =1

Molecular weight = Weight of imperial formula

Many methods employed for the determination of molecular weight of compounds viz.

1. Physical methods

(a) *For volatile compounds*

(i) Victor Meyer's method
(ii) Duma's method
(iii) Hofman's method

(b) *For non-volatile compounds*

(i) Ebullioscopic or elevation in boiling point method
 • Lands Berger's method
 • Cotterell's method

(ii) Cryoscopic or depression in freezing point method

- Beckmann's method
- Rast-camphor method

2. Chemical methods

(i)   Silver salt method
(ii) Platinic chloride method
(iii) Volumetric method for acid and base

3. Other methods

(i)   Osmatic pressure measurement method
(ii)   Viscosity measurement method
(iii) Light scattering method
(iv)   Diffusion method
(v)   Electrophoresis method
(vi)   Sedimentation method
(vii) X-ray analysis method
(viii) Chromatographic method
(ix)   Ultrafiltration method
(x)   Selective precipitation method

Colligative properties

The properties of solution containing non-volatile solute, which do not depend upon the nature of solute dissolved but depends upon the number of solute particles in solution are called as colligative properties such as

(a) Osmotic pressure $\pi \propto n$ where $\Delta \pi V = n. S .T$
(b) Lowering of the vapor pressure $\Delta P \propto n$ where $\Delta P / P_0 = n / (n + N)$
(c) Elevation of boiling point $\Delta T_b \propto n$ where $\Delta T_b = 1000 K_b.w / m \times W$

EXERCISE NO. 2.1

To determine molecular weight of volatile substance by Victor Meyer's Method

Purpose

- To learn method of determination of molecular weight of volatile substances.
- To study the factor effecting determination of molecular weight of the substance.

Requirements

Chemicals/Reagents

- Chloroform
- or acetone
- or methyl alcohol
- Distilled water

Equipments/Glasswares

- Victor Meyer's apparatus
- Hoffmann's bottle
- Gas burette
- Burette stands
- Glass jar
- Glass wool

Procedure

1. Arrange the apparatus as shown in the Fig. 2.1.
2. Put a small amount of glass wool or asbestos in the dried inner tube.
3. Fill water in out side jacket.
4. Using the rubber cork, place this tube slightly above the water jacket.
5. Dip a tube in the cork as shown in the fig. 2.1.
6. Fill small amount of liquid (0.1g) in a weighed Hoffmann's bottle.
7. Transfer this tube immediately into the inner tube carefully.
8. Liquid is vaporized spontaneously.
9. The vapor is formed which is displaces an equivalent amount of volume of air from inner tube.
10. When the bubbling siezes, open the stopper from the inner tube.
11. Measure the air displaced in the jar at room temperature.

12. Record the pressure using barometer.
13. Repeat this experiment two to three time.

Observations

1. Room temperature $\quad\quad\quad\quad\quad\quad\quad\quad$ = t °C
2. Atmospheric pressure $\quad\quad\quad\quad\quad\quad$ = P mm hg
3. Weight of empty Hoffmann bottle $\quad\quad$ = W_1 g
4. Weight of empty Hoffmann bottle + test solution = W_2 g
5. Volume of air $\quad\quad\quad\quad\quad\quad\quad\quad\quad$ = V ml
6. Aqueous tension of water at t °C $\quad\quad$ = p mm

Calculation

1. Weight of liquid taken = $(W_2 - W_1)$ g
2. Pressure of dry air $\quad$ = $(P - p)$ mm

Gaseous equation

$$\boxed{P_1V_1/T_1 = P_0V_0/T_0}$$ --- (2.1)

Calculate V_0

$$\boxed{V_0 = P_1V_1/T_1 \times T_0/P_0}$$ --- (2.2)

Where, $P_1 = (P - p)$ $\quad\quad$ $P_0 = 760$
$\quad\quad\quad\quad$ $V_1 = V$ $\quad\quad\quad\quad$ $T_0 = 273$
$\quad\quad\quad\quad$ $T_1 = t + 273$ $\quad\quad$ $V_0 = ?$

∴ Molecular weight of the substance = $22400 \times (W_2 - W_1) / V_0$

Result

The molecular weight of the given liquid = ----------------.

EXERCISE NO. 2.2

To estimate composition of a binary mixture of volatile liquids by Vector Meyer's method

Purpose

- To learn the method of determination of percent substance in the binary mixture.

Requirements
Chemicals/Reagents

- Two miscible volatile liquids

Equipments/Glasswares

Same as exercise no. 2.1

Procedure

1. Step 1 to 5 same as exercise no.2.1.
2. Fill small amount of binary mixture of liquids in a weighed Hoffmann's bottle.
3. Transfer this tube immediately into the inner tube carefully.
4. Liquid is vaporized spontaneously.
5. The vapor is formed which is displaces an equivalent amount of volume of air from inner tube.
6. When the bubbles is stop to come out open the stopper from the inner tube.
7. Measure the air displaced in the jar at room temperature.
8. Determine the vapor density of the binary mixture.
9. As step 2 to 7 repeat again using only single volatile substance in place of mixture which is one of the liquid of the binary composition.
10. In the same way determine vapor density of another liquid of binary mixture.

Observations

1. Room temperature   = t °C
2. Atmospheric pressure   = P mm hg
3. Weight of empty Hoffmann bottle   = W_1 g
4. Volume of air   = V ml
5. Aqueous tension of water at t °C   = p mm
6. Weight of empty Hoffmann bottle + test solution A   = W_A g
7. Weight of empty Hoffmann bottle + test solution B   = W_B g
8. Weight of empty Hoffmann bottle + binary mixture   = W_{AB} g

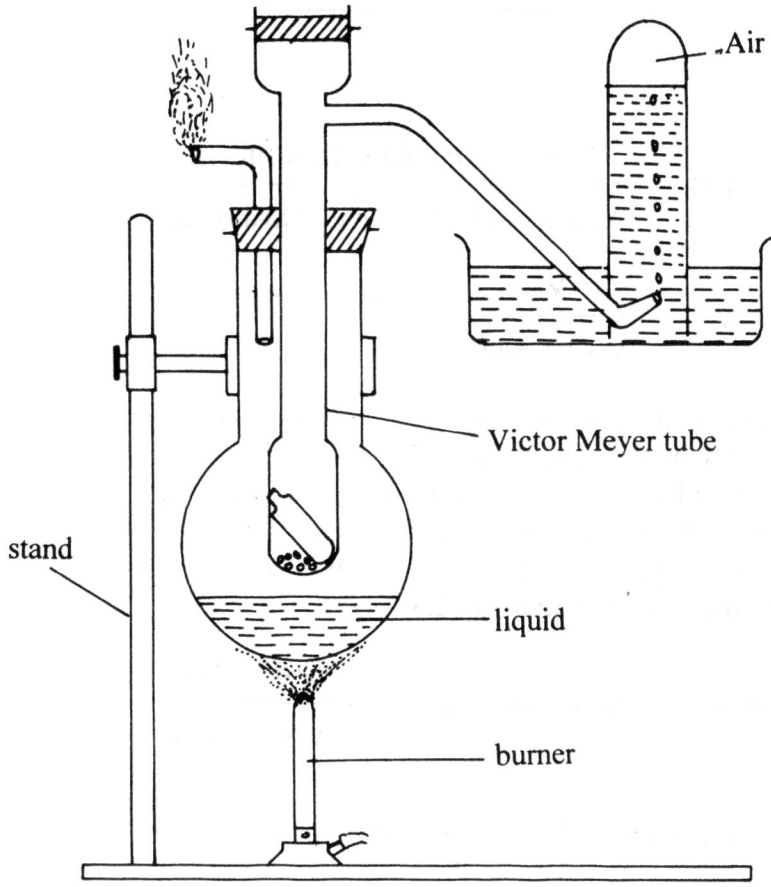

Fig. 2.1. Victor's Meyers apparatus

Calculation

1. Weight of liquid taken A   = $(W_A - W_1)$ g
2. Weight of liquid taken B   = $(W_B - W_1)$ g
3. Weight of binary liquids (AB) = $(W_A - W_1)$ g
4. Pressure of dry air   = $(P - p)$ mm

Gaseous equation

$$P_1 V_1 / T_1 = P_0 V_0 / T_0$$

Calculate V_A, V_B, and V_{AB} vapor densities of liquid A, liquid B and binary mixture of two liquids (AB) using the same way as exercise no.2.1.

$$V_0 = P_1V_1/T_1 \times T_0/P_0 \qquad \text{--- (2.3)}$$

Calculation

Vapor density   V.D. = $\dfrac{\text{Weight of certain volume of gas}}{\text{Weight of same volume of hydrogen}}$ $\qquad$ --- (2.4)

$$\text{V.D.} = \dfrac{W}{V \times 0.00009} \qquad \text{--- (2.5)}$$

(a) Vapor density of liquid A $\quad (d_A) = (W_A - W_1)/ V_A \times 0.00009$
$\quad$ V_A is determine by the equation no. 2.3

(b) Vapor density of liquid A $\quad (d_B) = (W_B - W_1)/ V_A \times 0.00009$
$\quad$ V_A is determine by the equation no. 2.3

(c) Vapor density of liquid A $\quad (d_{AB}) = (W_{AB} - W_1)/ V_A \times 0.00009$
$\quad$ V_A is determine by the equation no. 2.3

Weight of liquid A in binary mixture (w_A) = $w \times \dfrac{d_A(d_B - d_{AB})}{d_{AB}(d_B - d_A)}$

Composition of liquid A by weight = $\dfrac{w_A}{w} \times 100$

$$= w \times \dfrac{d_A(d_B - d_{AB})}{d_{AB}(d_B - d_A)} \qquad \text{--- (2.6)}$$

Calculate the composition of liquid B by weight = $w - w_A$
Determine the percent composition in the same as equation no. 2.6

Result

The binary mixture contains liquid A ----% and liquid B -----%.

EXERCISE NO. 2.3

To determine molecular weight of liquid by steam distillation method

Purpose

- To learn principle & method of determination of mol. weight by steam distillation.

Requirements

Chemicals/Reagents

- Toluene or nitrobenzene
- or aniline or benzene

Equipments/Glasswares

- Steam distillation apparatus
- Thermometer
- Graduated cylinder

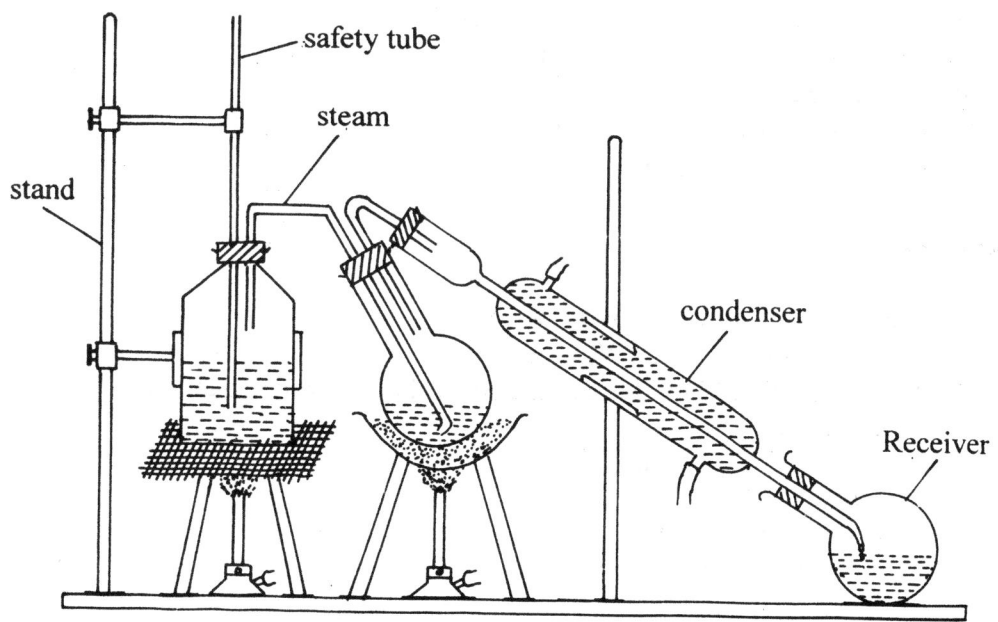

Fig. 2.2. Steam distillation apparatus

Procedure

1. Arrange the steam distillation apparatus as shown in the fig. 2.2.
2. Take mixture of liquids in round bottom flask. (containing 50 ml of liquid like aniline or toluene and 50 of distilled water).
3. Pass the steam from one container to the round bottom flask containing mixture of liquids and clamp at an angle.
4. Flask should be heated on sand bath so as to avoid condensation of water into the container.
5. Collect the distillate in the receiver.
6. About 10 ml of first distillate is to be rejected and then collect 35-40 ml of the distillate in receiver.

Observations

1. Volume of water collected $= V_w$ ml
2. Volume of liquid collected $= V_l$ ml
3. Temperature of distillation $= t$ °C
4. Atmospheric pressure $= P$ mm
5. Density of water (d_w) $= \text{-----}$ g/cm3
6. Density of liquid (d_l) $= \text{-----}$ g/cm^3
7. Density of liquid (d_l) $= \text{-----}$ g/cm^3
8. Molecular weight of water $= m_w$
9. Molecular weight of liquid $= m_l$
10. Vapor pressure of water $= p_w$
11. Vapor pressure of liquid (p_l) $= P - p_w$

Calculation

(a) Weight of liquid collected (W_l) $= d_l \times V_l$
(b) Weight of water collected (W_w) $= d_w \times V_w$
(c) Molecular weight of liquid is calculated by the following equation

$$m_A = \frac{W_l}{W_w} \times \frac{p_w \, m_w}{p_l}$$

Result

The molecular weight of the given liquid = ------------.

EXERCISE NO. 2.4

To determine molecular weight of non-volatile substance using water as solvent.

Purpose

- To learn principle of depression of freezing point of a liquid produced by dissolving a weighed amount of non-volatile solute in a known amount of the liquid.
- To study the factors affecting determination of the molecular weight.

Requirements

Chemicals/Reagents

- Glucose
- Urea
- Distilled water
- Ice

Equipments/Glasswares

- Beckmann's freezing point depression apparatus
- Thermometer
- Beckmann thermometer
- Stirrer

Procedure

1. Weigh accurately a 50 ml flask that is completely filled with distilled water.
2. Transfer 25 to 40 g of water, cover the bulb of the backmann thermometer and take weight again.
3. Prepare tablet of the substance using punching machine of weight about to 0.2 to 0.4 g.
4. Set the Bechmann thermometer as shown in Fig. 2.3.
5. Attach the Beckmann thermometer and stirrer to the inner tube.
6. Make freezing mixture tube using crushed ice and common salt.
7. Fill it in the glass jar surrounding the outer glass jacket.
8. Maintain the temperature through out the study.
9. Immerse the freezing tube having thermometer and stirrer directly into the freezing mixture.

10. Start the water stir slowly. Temperature falls rapidly when solid begins to separate.
11. Remove the freezing point tube from the bath and dry it, transfer it quickly in the outer glass jacket.
12. Stir continuously and record the temperature till it is constant. This is the freezing point of water.
13. Remove the inner tube from the outer glass jacket and melt the ice by rotating with the palm.
14. Replace it in the outer tube and now allow the temperature to decrease with constant stirring within a few seconds.
15. Now remove the inner tube and melt the ice.
16. Place an accurately weighed amount of tablet of the substance into the side tube.
17. Stir it well to dissolve the substance and consider all observation parameter as discussed.
18. Add further amounts of the solute and determine the freezing point.
19. Repeat the experiment for accuracy.

Observations

1. Weight of empty flask and distilled water = w_1 g
2. Weight of flask after transferring water = w_2 g
3. Weight of water used in freezing point = $w_1 - w_2$ g

Observation table

S.No.	Total weight of solute added (g)	Freezing point of solution	Freezing point mean	Depression of freezing point	Molecular weight
1.					
2.					
3.					
4.					
5.					

Calculation

Molecular weight of substance calculated by this equation

Molecular weight of substance (m) = 1000 K_w / ΔTW

Result

Molecular weight of the substance = ------------.

EXERCISE NO. 2.5

To determine molecular weight of a non-electrolyte substance using benzene as solvent

Purpose

- To learn method and principle for determination of molecular weight of non-electrolyte

Requirements

Chemicals/Reagents

- Benzene
- Camphor
- OR anthracene
- Or naphthalene
- Distilled water

Equipments/Glasswares

Same as exercise no. 2.4.

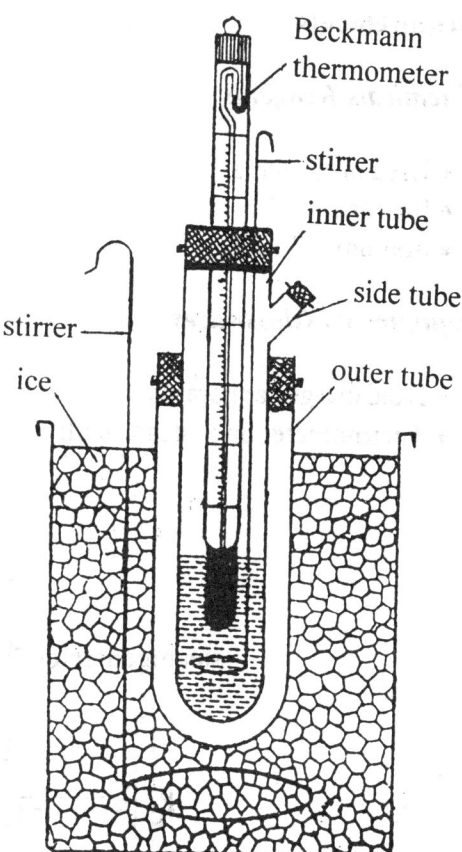

Fig. 2.3. Beckmann's apparatus

Labels: Beckmann thermometer, stirrer, inner tube, side tube, outer tube, stirrer, ice

Procedure

1. Arrange the assembly as shown in the fig. 2.3.
2. Set the Beckmann thermometer for freezing point of benzene about to 5.5 °C.
3. For maintaining this prepare mixture of pure ice and water in a beaker.
4. Fill the crushed ice in the cooling glass jar.
5. Determine the freezing points of benzene as exercise no. 2.4.
6. Calculate the molecular weight of the substance using the equation as given in exercise no. 2.4.

Observations & calculation

Same as exercise no. 2.4.

Result

The molecular weight of the given substance = ---------.

EXERCISE NO. 2.6

To determine molecular weight of a given substance by Landsberger method

Purpose

- To learn colligative properties of solutions and their importance.

Requirements

Chemicals/Reagents

- Urea or thiourea
- Sucrose
- Sodium chloride

Equipments/Glasswares

- Landsberger apparatus
- Thermometer and steam bath

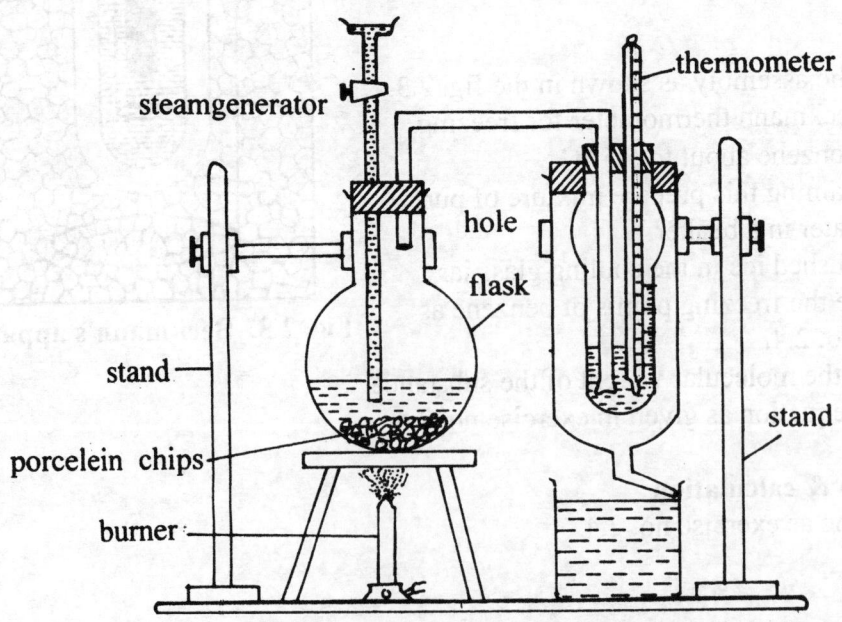

Fig. 2.4. Landsberger apparatus

Procedure

1. Set up the assembly as shown in fig. 2.4.
2. Take 10 ml of distilled water in the inner tube of the apparatus.
3. Produce steam from steam generation flask and pass into the Landsberger's apparatus inner tube.
4. Boiling point of the solvent is measured by the thermometer attached to the instrument.
5. Remove the water from the inner tube by disconnecting the rubber tube.
6. Weigh accurately 0.5 g of the substance and transfer in the inner tube and add 10 ml of distilled water in the inner tube.
7. Further attach the rubber tube and pass the steam.
8. Measure the boiling point of this solution by thermometer.
9. Stop supply of steam in the apparatus and cool this solution at room temperature.
10. Record the volume of the solution.
11. Calculate the weight of the solution in weight per ml of the substance.
12. Determine weight of solvent by substracting the weight of solute from the weight of solution.
13. Take different amounts of solute and repeat the experiment.
14. Molecular weight of the substance is determined by equation.

Observations

(a) Boiling point of pure solvent   = -- °C
(b) Density of solvent at room temperature = --- g/cm^3

Observation table

S.No.	Weight of solute added	Volume of solution	Boiling point of solution	Elevation of Boiling point ΔT	Molecular weight
1.					
2.					
3.					

Calculation

$$\text{Molecular weight of substance} = \frac{1000\ K_b\ w}{\Delta TW} = \frac{1000\ K_b\ w}{\Delta TVd}$$

Result

The molecular weight of the substance = ---------.

EXERCISE NO. 2.7

To determine molecular weight of a substance by Rast-Camphor method

Purpose

- To learn principle of freezing point or melting point of a pure compound.
- To learn principle of Rast-Camphor method for determination of molecular weight of the substance.

Requirements

Chemicals/Reagents

- Camphor
- Pure form of acetanilide and naphthalene
- Ether
- Resublimed sulphur

Equipments/Glasswares

- Melting point tube
- Thermometer
- Thin walled glass tube
- Capillary tubes

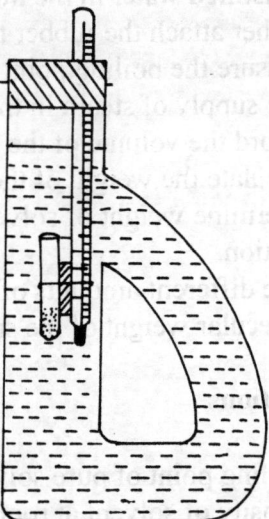

Fig. 2.5. Thiele's tube.

Procedure

1. Moisten the camphor using pure ether and reduce its particle size in an unglazed porcelain.
2. Take a small ignition tube and pull out its one end blowing off a small bulb and also close the other end after placing the powder inside the tube.
3. Determine the melting point of camphor.
4. Weigh accurate amount of camphor and acetanilide (about 10 times less than camphor) in an ampoule.
5. Seal this ampoule.
6. Melt the mixture by heating carefully.
7. Now cool the mixture at room temperature.
8. Break the ampoule and collect the material in closed petri plate.
9. Determine the melting point of mixture in the same way as step 1 to 3.
10. Calculate molecular weight by the datas obtained from the observation.

Observations

(a) Melting point of camphor = ------ °C

Observation table (A) for calibration

S.No.	Weight of camphor	Weight of solute	Melting point of solution				Depression of freezing point	K_f for camphor
			(a)	(b)	(c)	Mean		

Observation table (B) for molecular weight

S.No.	Weight of camphor	Weight of solute	Melting point of solution				Depression of freezing point	Molecular weight
			(a)	(b)	(c)	Mean		

Calculation

$$\text{Molecular weight of substance} = \frac{1000 \, K_b \, w}{\Delta TW} = \frac{1000 \, K_b \, w}{\Delta TVd}$$

Result

The molecular weight of the substance = ---------.

Viva-voce Question Bank

1. What is molecular weight of substances?
2. How to determine molecular weight of substance?
3. What are the factors affecting molecular weight?
4. What is the role of molecular weight of the substance?
5. Define vapor pressure of liquids.
6. How you can differentiate sodium chloride with urea.
7. Define colligative properties of solution.
8. Give principle involved in the determination of molecular weight by Landsburgers's method.
9. Define melting point.
10. Define freezing and boiling point of the substance.
11. Why are you determining the boiling point of the substance?
12. Give application of freezing point depression applicable in the field of pharmacy.

☐☐☐

Chapter 3

DENSITY OF LIQUIDS

Density is a derived quantity. It is defined as the mass per unit volume at a fixed temperature and pressure.
It can be determined using equation-

$$\text{Density} = \frac{\text{Weight}}{\text{Volume}}$$

Unit of density in CGS is g/cm^3 (grams per cubic centimeter). Number of terms are used to represents the mass or weight of equal volume of different substances e.g.
1. Absolute density
2. Apparent density
3. Relative density
4. Specific density

Absolute density : Absolute density is the ratio of mass of a substance to the volume of the substance at a specific temperature. (Mass of any substance is referred as the weight of substances at a specific temperature)

$$\text{Absolute density} = \frac{\text{Mass in grams (in a vacuum)}}{\text{Volume in milliliter}}$$

Apparent density : Apparent density is the ratio of mass of a substance in air to the volume of the substance at a specific temperature.

$$\text{Apparent density} = \frac{\text{Mass in grams (in air)}}{\text{Volume in milliliter}}$$

Relative density : Relative density is an expression, which exhibits mass of 1 ml of a standards substances such as water at a specific temperature, relative to water at 4°C temperature as unity.

At 4°C the relative density of water is 1.0000 and absolute density of water at same temperature is 0.999973. Relative density of water can be converted to absolute density by multiplying it by 0.99973.

Specific density : Specific density may be defined as the ratio of the mass of a substance to the mass of an equal volume of another substance taken as standards.

$$\text{Specific density} = \frac{Ws/V}{Ww/V} = \frac{Ws}{Ww}$$

where Ws – weight of substance, Ww – weight of equal volume of water and V – volume in milliliter.

The standard for gases may be taken as hydrogen or air; standards for liquids and solid may be taken as water. Specific gravity determination depends on the medium such as air or vacuum. If the specific gravity is determined in the vacuum, the result is a true specific gravity & is called as absolute specific gravity while the masses of the substance in air, is known as apparent specific gravity. According to USP and NF specific gravity is defined as,' the ratio of the weight of a substance in air at 25°C to that of an equal volume water at the same temperature.' It is not always necessary to determine the weight of substance and weight of water at the same temperature i.e. 25°C or any other temperature. It may be also possible that the substance may be weighed at 25°C and compared with that at 4°C. In this case the specific gravity is mentioned or reported as 25°/4°. In case of theobroma oil, which is, solid at 25°C, the specific gravity of the theobroma oil is determined on a 100°/25°bases and in case of alcohol, the specific gravity is determined on a 15.56°/15.56° bases because US government has adopted all the alcoholometric measurement at the same temperature i.e.60°F (15.56°C).

Specific gravity is the ratio of the weight of a substance in air to that of an equal volume of water hence it does not have any unit while gravity has units of mass over volume. In the metric system both density and specific gravity is numerically equal while density has units. In the English system, specific gravity and density are not numerically equal e.g. the density of water is 62.4 lb/ft^3 and specific gravity is one.

Instruments

Specific gravity may be determined by the use of various types of methods using different types of equipments, viz.

- Pycnometer
- Density bottle (specific gravity bottle)
- Mohr-Westphal balance
- Hydrometer
- Other devices

Generally pycnometer and density bottles are used for the determination of density, specific gravity or relative density in the laboratory.

Density bottle

Density bottle is made of glass, with 5-25 cm^3 capacity and capillary stopper fitted into its mouth as shown in Fig. 3.2.

Pycnometer

Pycnometer is made of glass having 10-25 cm^3 capacity. It consists of U-tube with a cylindrical bulb and two capillary arms (Fig. 3.1). Liquids are filled from one side arm (R) and sucked from the other end of the arm (P). It is a most convenient, accurate and economic apparatus for determination of density of liquids.

Volume

Volume is a measurable quantity. It is expressed in term of liter, ml, cubic centimeter etc. Volume of a 1g of water at 1 atmospheric pressure and 4°C was equivalent to 1 cc. 1 liter = 000.027 cm^3. There is a discrepancy between the milliliter and cubic centimeter but it is very small as to be disregarded in the general chemical and pharmaceutical practices. Volume in pharmaceutical practice is generally represented in ml (milliliter). Following apparatus are employed for the measurement of volume of liquids viz. Measuring cylinder

- Cylindrical and conical droppers
- Graduated pipette
- Simple pipette

- Burette
- Graduated droppers

Specific volume (V)

The volume occupied by 1 g of substance at a given temperature and pressure is called specific volume. It is equal to the reciprocal of density of the substance.

$$V = \frac{1}{\rho} \ cm^3/g$$

Molar Volume (Vm)

It is defined as the volume occupied by 1 g mole of the substance at a given temperature and pressure. Mathematically, it is determined by molecular weight divided by density of liquid.

$$Vm = \frac{Mw}{\rho}$$

where, Vm - molar volume, Mw – molecular weight of the substance and ρ - density of substance.

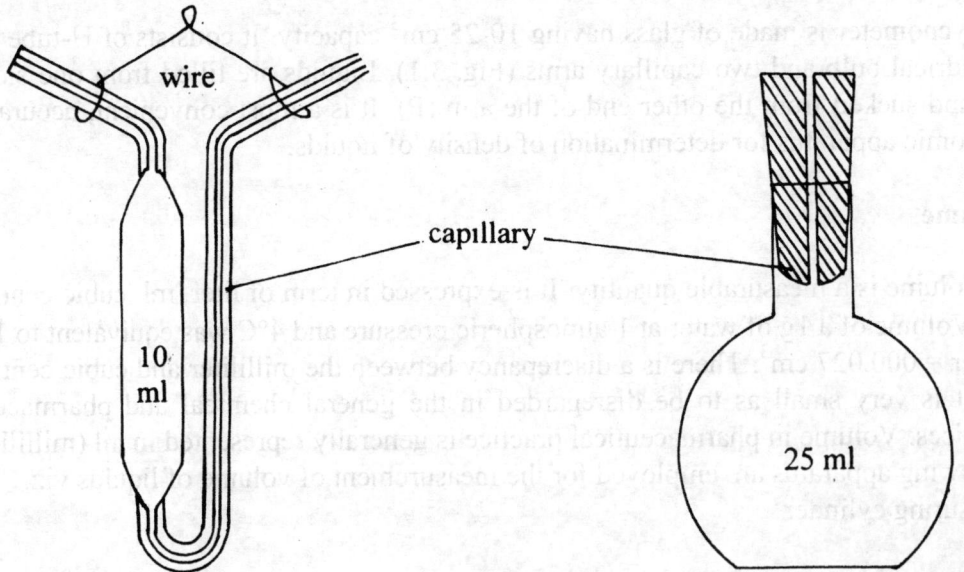

Fig. 3.1. Pycnometer .   Fig. 3.2. Density bottle with capillary stopper.

EXERCISE NO. 3.1

Determine density of water at different temperature using pycnometer

Purpose

- To learn concepts of density and its utility

Requirements

Chemicals/reagents
- Purified water

Equipments/glasswares

- Pycnometer
- Thermometer
- Beaker 100 ml, 250ml and 1 L.
- Burette stand
- Weight box
- Weighing balance

Procedure

1. Clean the pycnometer using chromic acid solution and then rinse with purified water. Rinse it using acetone and then dry it by current of air or using oven.
2. Hang the dry pycnometer with the help of platinum wire or copper wire to burette stand.
3. Weigh the dry pycnometer
4. Fill the pycnometer with distilled water by dipping one end of the capillary in distilled water. Suck the water carefully from another arm of the pycnometer.
5. Weigh the pycnometer with water.
6. Hang the filled pycnometer in the 1L flask containing water (temporary water bath)
7. Take the weight of pycnometer at different temperature after maintaining temperature($37°,42°,55°,68°,75°,85°$ and $95°$)
8. Repeat the experiment at least three times.

Observations

1. Volume of pycnometer $= V$ ml
2. Weight of empty and dry pycnometer $= W_1$ g
3. Weight of pycnometer with water $= W_2$ g

4. Weight of water in pycnometer $= W_2 - W_1$ g

Observation table

S.No.	Temperature (°C)	Weight of Pycnometer with water	Density of water (g/cm³)
1	Room	W_2	
2	temperature		
3	37		
4	42		
5	55		
6	68		
7	75		
8	85		
9	95		

Calculation*

Density of water at room temperature

$$\rho = \frac{\text{Weight of water at room temperature } (W2 - W1)}{\text{Volume of pycnometer } (V)}$$

Result

Report the result on the bases of calculation of density. (Density of water decreases with the increasing of temperature).

It is important in case of water. Density of water is highest i.e. 1.0 at 4°C. While increase in temperature (above 4°C) and decreasing (below 4°C) of temperature of water, density decreases.

---

*Calculate density of water at different temperature by the equation no-1. Plot the graph between temperature and density.

EXERCISE NO. 3.2

Determine density of given liquid at a definite temperature using
(a) Density bottle   (b) Pycnometer

Purpose

- To learn determination of density by density bottle and pycnometer.

Requirements

Chemicals/reagents

- Sucrose solution or calamine lotion or octanol or castor oil
- Liquid paraffin or
- 2% solution of sodium salicylate

Equipments/glasswares

- Pycnometer
- Density bottle
- Themometer
- Beaker 100 ml, 250ml
- Burette stand
- Weight box
- Weighing balance

Procedure

1. Thoroughly clean the density bottle and pycnometer with chromic acid or ntric acid.
2. Rinse the density bottle and pycnometer with purified water two to three times.
3. If necessary rinse and dry using organic solvents like methanol,acetone etc.
4. Take weight of dry density bottle with stopper (Capillary tube).
5. Fill the bottle with the purified water and place the stopper. Small amount of water comes out by the capillary, wipeout the excess liquid out side the tube using tissue paper.
6. Weigh the density bottle with water using balance.
7. After removing the water, rinse the density bottle with the liquid and fill the liquid in the density bottle in the same way.
8. Weigh the density bottle with testing liquid.
9. Repeat the experiment at least three times and report average on the record book.

10. Apply same method as mentioned in the experiment no.1 for determination of density by pycnometer.

Observations

1. Volume of density bottle = V ml
2. Weight of empty and dry density bottle with stopper = W_1 g
3. Weight of density bottle with water = W_2 g
4. Weight of density bottle with testing liquid = W_3 g
5. Weight of water in density bottle = $W_2 - W_1$ g
6. Weight of testing liquid in density bottle = $W_3 - W_1$ g
7. Volume of pycnometer = V' ml
8. Weight of empty and dry pycnometer = W'_1 g
9. Weight of pycnometer with water = W'_2 g
10. Weight of pycnometer with testing liquid = W'_3 g
11. Weight of water in pycnometer = $W'_2 - W'_1$ g
12. Weight of testing liquid in pycnometer = $W'_3 - W'_1$ g

Calculation

1. Density of liquid determined by density bottle at temperature t°C or room temperature.

$$\text{Density of liquid at t °C or room temperature} = \frac{\text{Weight of liquid at t °C} (W'_3 - W_1)}{\text{Weight of water at t °C} (W_2 - W_1)} \times \text{Density of water at t °C}$$

2. Density of liquid determined by pycnometer at temperature t°C or room temperature.

$$\text{Density of liquid at t °C or room temperature} = \frac{\text{Weight of liquid at t °C} (W'_3 - W'_1)}{\text{Weight of water at t °C} (W'_2 - W'_1)} \times \text{Density of water at t°C}$$

Result

Density of liquid = ------ g/cm^3 determined by density bottle at t °C and density of liquid = ------ g/cm^3 determined by pycnometer at t °C.

EXERCISE NO. 3.3

To study the effect of temperature on density of given liquid using pycnometer

Purpose
- learn the effect of temperature on density.

Requirements

Chemicals/reagents

- Sucrose solution or calamine lotion or octanol or castor oil
- Liquid paraffin or
- 2% solution of sodium salicylate

Equipments/glasswares
Same as exercise no. 3.1

Procedure

1. Hang the pycnometer in water bath or in beaker (1 liter).
2. Follow the same procedure as mentioned in the experiment no. 3.1

Observation
Same as exercise no. 3.1

Observation table

S.No.	Temperature (°C)	Weight of pycnometer		Average weight (a +b)	Density (calculated)
		Increasing order(a)	Decreasing order (b)		

Result

Density of the liquid increases/decreases with the increasing of temperature.
(Plot the graph between temperature and density).

Note : Compare the density obtained by using two apparatus and study the main cause of the difference of the densities while other physical parameters are same. If there is major difference repeat the experiment at least three times and discuss with the teacher for major causes of differences in the densities.

EXERCISE NO. 3.4

To study the effect of temperature on density of given liquid using density bottle

Purpose

- To learn the effect of temperature on density using density bottle.

Requirements

Chemicals/reagents

- Sucrose solution or calamine lotion or octanol or castor oil
- Glycerin
- Liquid paraffin

Equipments/glasswares
    Same as exercise no. 3.2
Procedure

1. Follow step 1to 6 as exercise no. 3.2
2. Put the liquid in water bath or hot plate for raising the temperature and maintain the temperature till 5 min.
3. Fill the density bottle with liquid at particular temperature. It is necessary to take at least 2-5 °C more than the study temperature because density bottles as well as in the handling procedure affects the temperature.
4. Other steps are same as mentioned in the Experiment No-1.3.

Observation
    Same as exercise no. 3.2

Observation Table

S.No.	Temperature (°C)	Weight of density bottle		Average weight (a +b)	Density (calculated)
		Increasing order (a)	Decreasing order (b)		

Result
    Density of the liquid increases/decreases with the increasing of temperature.
(Plot the graph between temperature and density).

EXERCISE NO. 3.5

To study the effect of salt viz., sodium chloride in different concentration on the density of water at 25°C or room temperature.

Purpose

- To study the effect of addition of salt on density.
- To make understand the students with change in the density due to addition of sodium chloride and develop the concept for the determination of concentration of the sodium chloride in the unknown solution on the basis of density concept using pycnometer or density bottle at define temperature or room temperature or at 25°C

Requirements

Chemicals/reagents

- Different concentration of sodium chloride in purified water(1-15%)
- Distilled water

Equipments/glasswares

- Pycnometer
- Thermometer
- Burette stand
- Beaker 100 ml, 250ml
- Weight box
- Weighing balance

Procedure

1. Prepare 1%, 2%, --------10% solution of sodium chloride in purified water at room temperature each about to 50 ml.
2. Fill these solution in the reagent bottle.
3. If any turbidity or impurities in the solution, filter it or prepare fresh solution because any type of impurities varies result .
4. Follow all steps exercise no. 3.1.
5. Record the weight at least four decimal value.
6. Determine the density of the different concentration the solutions as performed in step two.

Observations

1. Volume of pycnometer $= V$ ml
2. Weight of empty and dry pycnometer $= W_1$ g
3. Weight of pycnometer with water $= W_2$ g

Observation Table

S.No.	Concentration of NaCl in purified water (% w/v)	Weight of Pycnometer			Average weight (a +b+c)	Density (Calculated)
		a	b	c		
1	0					
2	1					
3	2					
-	-					
-	-					
11	10					

Result

Calculate the density of the liquid at different concentration as per procedure given in experiment no 1.2.

Plot the graph between concentration and density. On the basis of graph determine the density of unknown sample of the same liquid.

EXERCISE NO. 3.6

To prepare different concentration of sucrose in purified water and determine density at room temperature using density bottle and pycnometer.

Purpose

- To study the effect of salt in different concentration on density.
- To make understand the students change in the density with increase in the concentration of sucrose solution using pycnometer or density bottle at definite temperature or room temperature or at 25 °C

Requirements

Chemicals/reagents

- Different concentration of sucrose in purified water(1-15%)
- Sucrose
- Purified water

Equipments/glasswares

- Pycnometer
- Density bottle
- Beaker 100 ml, 250ml
- Weight box
- Weighing balance

Procedure

1. Prepare 1%, 2%, --------10% solution of sucrose in purified water at room temperature each about to 50 ml.
2. Determine the density of the prepared sucrose solution at room temperature using density bottle and pycnometer as exercise no 3.5.

Result

Calculate the density of the liquid at different concentration as per procedure given in experiment no 3.2.
Plot the graph between concentration and density. On the basis of graph, determine the density of unknown sample of the same liquid.

EXERCISE NO. 3.7

To prepare different composition of glycerin and water and determine density at room temperature. (For accuracy provide unknown samples)

Purpose
- To learn the effect of diluting a solution on density at room temperature

Requirements

Chemicals/reagents

- Different compotion of glycerin and purified water
- Glycerin

Equipments/glasswares
    Same as exercise no. 3.1

Procedure

1. Prepare different composition of glycerin & purified water 10:90, 20:80, 30:70, 40:60, 50:50, 60: 40, 70:30, 80:20 and 90:10 at room temperature each 50 ml.
2. Determine densities as exercise no. 3.6.
3. In the same way determine the density of the different composition.

Observation

Observation Table

S.No.	Different composition of glycerin and water	Weight of Pycnometer			Average weight (a +b+c)	Density (Calculated)
		a	b	c		
1	10:90					
2	20:80					
3	30:70					
4	40:60					
5	50:50					
6	60:40					
7	70:30					
8	80:20					
9	90:10					

Result

    Density of different composition increases/decreases with the increasing concentration of glycerin. (Plot the graph between concentration and density)

EXERCISE NO. 3.8

Determine the molal volume of ethanol at 25°C or room temperature.

Purpose

- To familiars the students with determination of molal volume and its importance.

Requirements

Chemicals/reagents

- Ethanol
- Distilled water

Equipments/glasswares

- Pycknometer
- Thermostat
- Thermameter
- Beaker 100 ml and 250 ml
- Weight box
- Weighing balance
- Other glasswares

Procedure

1. Prepare different composition of ethanol and water such as-10:90, 20:80, 30:70, 40:60, 50:50, 60: 40, 70:30, and 80:20 (%w/w) of ethanol, weigh accurately in the closed container or weighing bottle.
2. Determine the density of pure ethanol and different composition by adopting same method as mentioned in the Experiment no 1.6 at room temperature.
3. Calculate density of different composition as exercise no.3.1

Observations

(a) Volume of pycnometer	=	V ml
(b) Weight of empty pycnometer	=	W_1
(c) Weight of pycnometer + distilled water	=	W_2
(d) Molecular weight of ethanol	=	46.07

Observation Table

S.No.	Different composition of Ethanol & water (w/w)	Weight of Pycnometer			Average weight (a +b+c)	Density (Calculated)
		a	b	c		
1	10:90					
2	20:80					
3	30:70					
4	40:60					
5	50:50					
6	60:40					
7	70:30					
8	80:20					

Calculation

(a) Density of liquid calculated as exercise no. 3.1.

(b) Molal volume

$$V_m = \frac{\text{Molecular weight}}{\text{Density}}$$

(c) Specific volume is reciprocal of the density. Calculate the specific volume all compositions,

Result

Density of different composition -------------------&----- g/cm^3. Plot percentage by weight of ethanol against the specific volume. Draw a smooth curve and draw tangents to the curve at different concentrations.

Viva-voce Question Bank

1. What is density?
2. What is difference between density and specific gravity?
3. What is the importance of density in pharmaceutical formulation?
4. Give two examples of dosage form based on the density concepts.
5. Give factors affecting density.
6. What is effect of temperature on density?
7. What is the effect of concentration on density?
8. What is the density of water at 4°C?
9. What is temperature at which water has highest density?
10. Why are you studying density?
11. How to determine density?
12. How to use pycnometer?
13. Give advantages and disadvantages of pycnometer.
14. What is molar volume?
15. What is difference between cc and ml?

❐❐❐

Chapter 4

RHEOLOGY

The term rheology is suggested by Bingham and Crowford. It is a Greek word, formed from rheo (flow) and logus (science) which deals with deformation and flow matter. Rheology is involved in many fields such as circulation of fluid, flow of mucus, bending of bones, stretching of cartilage, contraction of muscle, flow of suspension, paints, inks, doughs, road building materials, cosmetics, dairy products, lotions, emulsion, syrup. Flow characteristics of semisolid formulation highly affect mixing and flow of materials.

Rheology play an important role in the various pharmaceutical products e.g. mixing, flow of materials, packaging into containers and their transfer prior to use, i.e. when these substances are transferred by pouring from a bottle, extrusion from a tube or passage through a syringe needle.

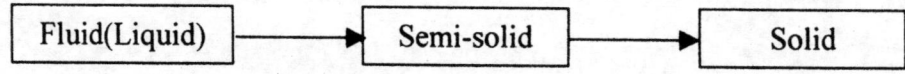

Fig 4.1. Range of Consistence.

Rheology can affect many parameters such as-
- Patient acceptability
- Physical stability
- Biological availability
- Syringeability
- Extrudability
- Pourability
- Flowability

Viscosity is a representation of the resistance of a fluid to flow and higher is the viscosity greater is the resistance. On the basis of flow and deformation, material can be classified mainly to category

1. Newtonian flow
2. Non-Newtonian flow

Newtonian flow

Fluids which follow Newton's law of flow is known as fluid having Newtonian flow. It states that 'the rate of shear is directly proportional to the shearing stress'. Let us consider a block as shown in rig. 4.2. If bottom layer is considered to be fixed and top plane of liquid is moved at a constant velocity. The rate of shear is directly proportional to the distance from the stationary bottom layer.

Velocity gradient or rate of shear = dv/dr

where, dv is velocity between two planes of liquids, dr is very small distance between two planes.

The force per unit area required to bring about flow is called the shearing stress.

Shearing stress = Force/Area = F'/A

According to Newtonian law

Shearing stress ∝ rate of shear
F'/A ∝ dv/dr
F'/A = η dv/dr

where η is called as coefficient of viscosity. It is generally represented in term viscosity. Viscosity or internal friction is the resistance to the relative motion of adjacent layer of liquid.

If use, F'/A = F and dv/dr = G Then η = F / G
If plot a graph between F & G it shows a
Straight line which passes through origin

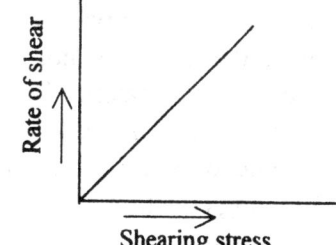

Fig. 4.2. Newtonian flow

Units and dimension of viscosity

Unit is in CGS unit- poise, small unit centipoise (10^{-2} poise).
Dimension of viscosity $[ML^{-1}T^{-1}]$

Fluidity : It is reciprocal of the viscosity

$$\phi = 1 / \eta$$ where, ϕ is the fluidity

Kinematic viscosity

Kinematic viscosity of a liquid is obtained when viscosity of the material is divided by the density of the same material in the similar state.

$$\text{Kinematic Viscosity (KV)} = \eta / \rho$$

The unit of kinematic viscosity is stoke(s) and centistoke (cs)

Non-Newtonian flow

Non-Newtonian flows fail to follow Newtonian equation of law. This flow can be divided in three categories
- Plastic flow
- Pseudoplastic flow
- Dilatant flow

Plastic flow

The plastic flow curve does not pass through the origin. The shearing stress axis at a definite point, shows a yield value. The yield value is important property of certain dispersion. The slope in the graph is termed as mobility (Shown in Fig. 4.3).

$$\text{Plastic viscosity} = \frac{F - f}{G}$$

where 'f' is the yield value. It is related with the pressure of the flocculated particle in concentrated suspensions. The yield value exhibits because of the contracts between adjacent particles. The yield value also shows the force of flocculation. If the suspension is more flocculated then the yield value is also higher.

Pseudoplastic Flow

Many pharmaceutical products such as liquid dispersion of tragacanth, sodium alginate, methylcellulose and sodium carboxymethylcellulose exhibits pseudoplastic flow. Polymer in the form of solution generally exhibits pseudoplastic flow. The consistency curve passes through the origin (Fig. 4.3). In this figure, as there is no yield value, the curve is not linear. Hence it is very difficult to determine viscosity of pseudoplastic material by using single value. The viscosity of pseudoplastic substance decreases with increase in the rate of shear. An apparent viscosity can be estimated at any rate of shear from the slope of tangent to the curve at a specific point by the following equation

$$F^N = \eta' G$$

Taking log both side

$$N \log F = \log \eta' + \log G$$

or

$$\log G = N \log F - \log \eta'$$

This is an equation for a straight line of many pseudoplastic systems follow this equation.

Dilatant Flow

Some suspension has high percent of dispersed solid and exhibit an increase in resistance to flow with increase in the rates of shear. In this system volume is increased with shear and is known as a dilatant flow. These types of flows just opposite to the pseudoplastic flow. Pseudoplastic materials generally contribute as " shear-thinning system" while dilatant materials contribute for "shear-thickening systems". When stress is removed from the dilatant system it regains original state of fluidty.

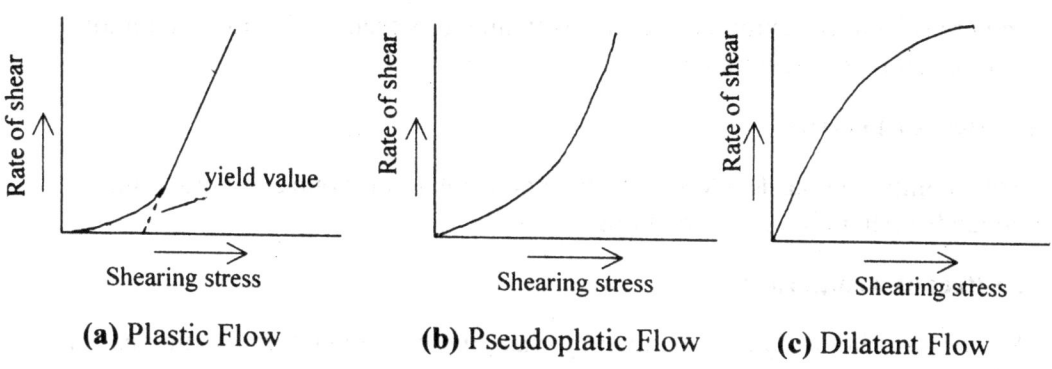

(a) Plastic Flow **(b)** Pseudoplatic Flow **(c)** Dilatant Flow

Fig. 4.3. Non-Newtonian Flow

Rheochor

It is a constant given by Newton Fried. It is the product of molar volume and eighth root of the coefficient of the viscosity and independent of temperature. This constant is called rheochor determined by the following equation

$$\text{Rheochor} = \frac{M\,\eta^{1/8}}{d}$$

where, d is the density, M is the molecular weight of the material, and η is the viscosity of the liquid.

Molecular Viscosity

Molecular viscosity is the product of viscosity and molecular surface.

Molecular viscosity = Molecular surface × Viscosity

$$\text{Molecular viscosity} = (M/d)^{2/3} \times \eta$$

Factor Effecting Viscosity

1. Effect of Molecular Weight

If molecular weight is increased using similar category of the substance, viscosity increases.

2. Branching of Organic Compounds

Most of the straight chain compounds have less viscosity than the branched chain compound.

3. Presence of Impurities

Impure substances exibits more viscosity due to presence of solutes, colloidal substances and other substances.

4. Effect of Polarity

Polar compound has less viscosity than non-polar compound because polar compounds contain hydrogen bonding.

5. Effect of Temperature

Viscosity of liquid can be changed by changing of temperature. Arrhenius equation is based on the same principle.

$$\eta = A e^{E/RT}$$

or $$\ln \eta = \ln A + E/RT$$

or $$2.303 \log \eta = 2.303 \log A + E/RT$$

or $$\log \eta = \log A + E/2.303 RT$$

where, A is a constant, E is the activation energy for viscous flow, R is the gas constant. Large value of E shows that the viscosity decreases with rise in the temperature.

Determination of Viscosity

Varieties of viscometer are commercially available for the determination of viscosity. It is necessary to select suitable viscometer according to the nature of the material. Viscometers are based on the three basic principles.

1. Measurement of viscosity is based on the rate of flow of a liquid through an orifice or a duct of simple geometry.
2. Resistance to rotation of a metallic body in contact with or immersed in the liquid.

3. Velocity of a metal sphere rolling or falling through the liquid under the effect of gravity or of an air bubble rising because of its limited use. Principle of this method is based on the Stoke's law.

$$v = \frac{2r^2(\rho - \rho_0)g}{9\eta_0}$$

where, v is velocity of spherical ball moving in the liquid of viscosity η_0, ρ, and ρ_0 are density of ball and liquid respectively and r is the radius of the ball. This equation is known as Stoke's equation.

Viscometers used for determination of viscosity of liquids and semisolids are

1. Capillary Viscometer
2. Falling Sphere Viscometer
3. Cup and Bob Viscometer
4. Cone and Plate Viscometer
5. Brookfield Synchro-Lectric Viscometer
6. Stormer Viscometer
7. Coaxial-Cylinder Viscometer
8. MacMichael Viscometer
9. Couette Viscometer
10. Haake Rotovisco Viscometer

Capillary Viscometer

The glass capillary Cannon-Fenske, Ubbehde and Ostwald viscometers are the most popular apparatus based on the first principle of flow of a liquid through an orifice or a duct of simple geometry. Ostwald viscometer consists of a cylindrical capillary tube and the driving force causing the liquid to flow through it is its weight. Poiseuille a French Physician studied the flow of liquids through capillary tubes and established a mathematical expression.

$$\frac{V}{t} = \frac{\pi r4 \Delta p}{8l\eta}$$

where, V/t is the rate of flow of liquid or flow in the capillary, Δ p represents the hydrostatic pressure of a liquid column of height h and density of liquid as d and g represents the acceleration of gravity.

$$\Delta p = h d g$$

$$\eta = \frac{\pi r4 t \Delta p}{8l V}$$

Poiseuille's equation

$$\eta = \frac{\pi r^4 \, t \, h \, d \, g}{8l \, V}$$

If instrumental constant

$$K = \frac{\pi r4 \, h \, g}{8l \, V}$$

Then $\eta = K \, t \, d$

It is not necessary to evaluate K. If two liquid A and B are considered having viscosities η_1 & η_2 and density d_1 and d_2 and time taken by them to flow between two fixed points is t1& t_2 respectively then it can be expressed as equation.

$$\eta_1 = K \, t_1 \, d_1 \quad \text{(i)} \qquad\qquad \eta_2 = K \, t_2 \, d_2 \quad \text{(ii)}$$

Equation (i) is divided by (ii)

$$\frac{\eta_1}{\eta_2} = \frac{t_1 \, d_1}{t_2 \, d_2} \quad \text{or} \quad \boxed{\eta_1 = \frac{t_1 \, d_1 \, \eta_2}{t_2 \, d_2}}$$

A range of glass capillary viscometer with different diameter are available for liquid of different viscosity.

Precautions
1. Instrument should be completely cleaned using chromic acid solution and if necessary then organic solvents like methanol or acetone.
2. Capillary diameter should be selected on the basis of viscosity of liquid.
3. For accuracy, take readings in triplicate.
4. A range of shear rates can be covered when external pressure is applied to force a viscous liquid through a narrow capillary.

Falling sphere viscometer

This type of viscometer consists of a glass tube & steel ball rolls. It moves vertically in the glass tube containing the test liquid at a control temperature. The rate of ball at which it moves in a fixed diameter tube is inversely proportional to the viscosity of liquids. If the viscosity of the liquids is high, ball is moved slowly in the liquid.

It is based on the principle that resistance offered by a liquid to falling ball is equal to its viscosity. Thus, velocity of the ball is inversely proportional to the viscosity. It consists of a ball placed in the inner glass tube which has the homogeneous temperature maintained by constant water jacket. The time for the ball to fall between two fixed points is accurately measured and experiment is repeated for several times. The viscosity of the liquid is calculated by the following equation

$$\eta = t\ (S_b - S_f)\ B$$

where, t is the time interval between two points in sec, S_b specific gravity of ball, S_f specific gravity of fluid medium and B is a constant for a particular ball and is supplied by the manufacturer. This instrument is suitable to measure the viscosity in the range 0.5-2,00,000 poise. For accuracy it is better to move the ball between two point not less than 30 seconds.

Cup and Bob viscometer

In cup and bob viscometer the sample liquid is sheared in the space between the outer wall of a bob and the inner wall of a cup into which bob fits. Many viscometer are based on the principle of cup and bob viscometer like-MacMichael viscometer, Searle-type viscometer, Rotovisco-viscometer, Stormer viscometer. This viscometer is not suitable to determine the viscosity less than 20 cps.
Rotational Viscometer follows this equation

$$\Omega = [(1/\ \eta)\ (T/4\pi h)] \times [(1/\ R_b{}^2 - 1/\ R_c{}^2)]$$

where, Ω is the angular viscosity in radius sec^{-1}, T is the torque in dynes cm, h is the depth to which bob is immersed in the liquid. R_b and R_c are the radius of bob and cup respectively.

Cone and plate viscometer

Cone and Plate viscometer consists of a rotating cone with a very obtuse angle and a stationary lower plate. The plate is slightly raised so that the cone just touches to the surface. The liquid is filled between triangular gap in cone and plate. The plate is adjusted at a constant temperature by water jacket or circulating water. The cone is driven at controlled speeds that can be varied continuously.
The viscous drag on the rotating cone, which exerts a force on a dynamometer, that is proportional to the shear stress. The angle θ formed by cone and plate is usually less than 3^0 and the average gap width is less than 2 mm. hence rate of shear is uniformly distributed. The viscosity is determined by the following equation-

$$\eta = [(3\ \theta/2\pi\ R_b{}^3)\ /\ (T/\ \Omega)]$$

where, T is the torque and Ω is the angular velocity and R_b is the maximum cone radius.
The amount of sample required is very small as compared to other instruments and plug flow problem is absent in this viscometer.

Brookfield Synchro- Lectric viscometer

This interment consists of 4 to 8 rotating spindles in the liquid placed in a beaker. The rate of shear various widely through out the sample. Each instrument has a set of interchangeable cylindrical spindles or discs of different diameter, to be used for liquids of different viscosities. The spindle is rotated using a synchronous motor by a beryllium-copper torsion spring. Different models of viscometer have springs of different degree of stiffens and suitable for different viscosity ranges. The degree to which the spring is twisted is shown by a pointer. Viscosity of liquid is determined by the multiplication of dial reading and spindle number with speed at which it is moving (This value is given in the specification, provided by the manufacturer). Viscosity is presented in the form of poise or centipoise.

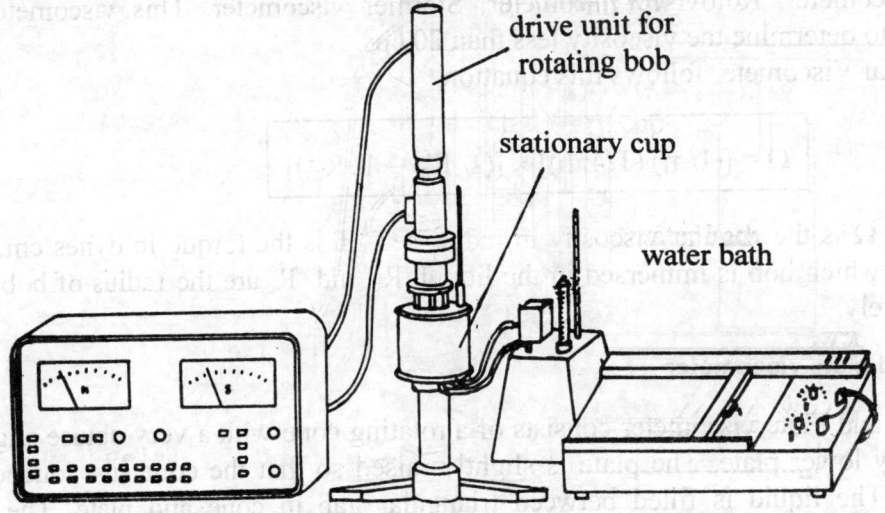

Fig. 4.4a . Haake rotovisco viscometer

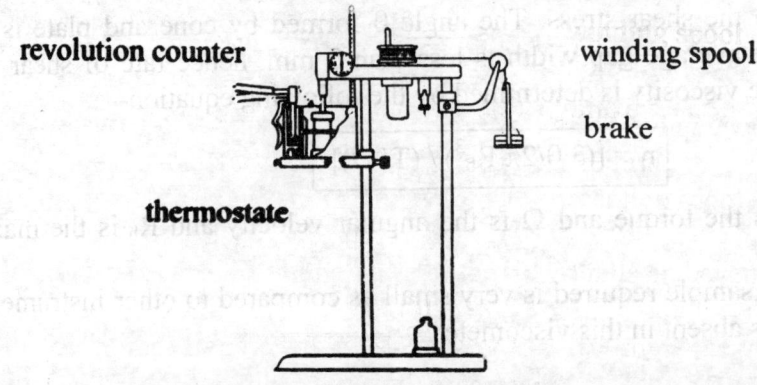

Fig. 4.4 b. Stormer viscometer

EXERCISE NO. 4.1

To determine viscosity of liquid using Ostwald's viscometer at room temperature

Purpose

- To study the flow characteristics of liquid and determine resistance to flow.
- To develop concept related to the viscosity and handling of viscometer.

Requirements

Chemicals/reagents

- Glycerin
- Or ethylacetate
- Or nitroglycerine
- Or cough syrup
- Or solutions
- Or simple syrup
- Distilled water
- Washing solution

Equipment /glasswares

- Ostwald's viscometer
- Pycnometer/density bottle
- Beaker
- Thermometer
- Burette stand
- Electronic balance
- Stopwatch
- Glassmarker
- Conical flask

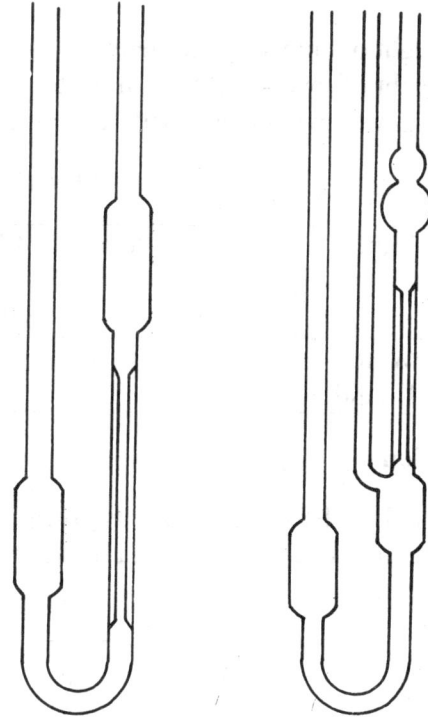

Fig. 4.5. Ostwald's viscometer.

Procedure

1. Thoroughly clean the viscometer with a mixture of warm chromic acid and if necessary clean the viscometer with solvent.
2. After cleaning the viscometer dry it completely by passing current of air or dry in the oven.
3. Fix the viscometer on the burette stand vertically.
4. Determine the density by pycnometer (as exercise no. 3.1).
5. Fill the purified water in the viscometer.
6. Report the time taken to flow water between two points.

7. Repeat the reading at least three times carefully and take average of these reading for calculation.
8. Remove purified water from the viscometer and rinse with the liquid under investigation for two to three times and then fill the liquid in the same way as purified water.
9. Further arrange the equipment properly and report the time taken to flow of liquid between two points A and B.
10. Take reading at least three times and take average of these readings for the calculation.

Observation

(a) Weight of empty pycnometer $\qquad$ = -----g
(b) Weight of pycnometer with water $\qquad$ = -----g
(c) Weight of pycnometer with testing liquid $\qquad$ = -----g

Observation Table

S.No.	Liquid	Time Taken to Flow of Liquid between two points (sec.)			Average (a+b+c)/3 (sec.)
		I (a)	II (b)	III (c)	
1	Water				
2	Liquid				

Calculation

(a) Calculate density of liquid as given in exercise no.3.1
(b) Calculate viscosity of liquid using the following formula

$$\eta_1 = \frac{t_1 d_1}{t_2 d_2} \times \eta_2$$

where,

- η_1 viscosity of liquid-----?
- η_2 viscosity of purified water at temperature (--°C).
- d_2 density of purified water at temperature (--°C).
- d_1 density of liquid calculated ---?
- t_1 flow time of liquid between two fixed point (taken from observation table).
- t_2 flow time of water between two fixed point (taken from observation table).

Result

Viscosity of given liquid (name of liquid) at room temperature (--°C) was -----------
poise or centipoise (cps), determine by Ostwald viscometer (Manufactured by---)

EXERCISE NO. 4.2

To determine viscosity of liquid using falling ball viscometer

Purpose

- To study the rate of ball through the testing liquid and develop concept /principle of viscosity.
- To develop concept related to the viscosity and handling of falling ball viscometer.

Requirements

Chemicals/reagents

- Glycerin
- or ethyl acetate
- or nitroglycerine
- or simple syrup
- Distilled water
- Washing solution

ball in
sample tube

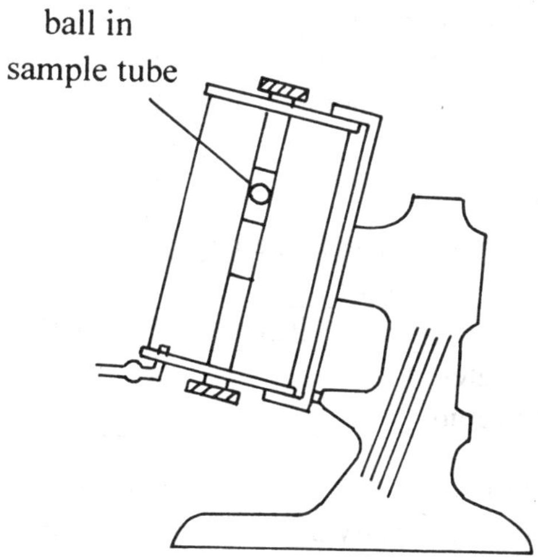

Fig. 4.6. Falling ball viscometer

Equipment /glasswares

- Pycnometer
- Beaker
- Thermometer
- Electronic balance
- Stopwatch
- Glassmarker
- Falling ball viscometer
- Conical flask

Procedure

1. Thoroughly clean the viscometer with a mixture of warm chromic acid and if necessary clean with solvent.
2. After cleaning the viscometer, dry it completely or rinse with the purified water two to three times.
3. Determine the viscosity using pycnometer (as exercise no. 3.1).
4. Fill purified water in the viscometer in the tube and close it properly.
5. Select the ball on the basis of viscosity of testing liquid.
6. Take time carefully of moving the ball from one point to another point as mentioned in the instrument.

7. Repeat the reading at least three time carefully and take average of these reading for calculation.
8. Transfer purified water from the viscometer and rinse with testing liquid two to three times and then fill the liquid in the same way as purified water (step 4).
9. Further arrange the equipment properly as step 5&6.
10. Note down the time carefully to move same ball between two points as mentioned in the instrument.
11. Take reading at least three consider and take average of these readings for the calculation.

Observation

(a) Temperature (Room Temperature)   =----- °C
(b) Weight of empty pycnometer   = -----g
(c) Weight of pycnometer with water   = -----g
(d) Weight of pycnometer with testing liquid = -----g

Observation Table

S.No.	Liquid	Time taken by ball to move between two points (sec.)			Average (a+b+c)/3 (sec.)
		I(a)	II(b)	III(c)	
1	Water				
2	Liquid				

Calculation
(a) Calculate density of liquid as given in exercise no. 3.1
(b) Calculate viscosity of liquid using the following formula

$$\eta_1 = \frac{t_1 d_1}{t_2 d_2} \times \eta_2$$

Where,
- η_1 viscosity of liquid-----?
- η_2 viscosity of purified water at temperature(--°C).
- d_2 density of purified water at temperature(--°C).
- d_1 density of liquid calculated ---?
- t_1 Time taken to move of ball in testing liquid between two fixed point (taken from observation table)
- t_2 Time taken to move the ball in purified water between two fixed point (taken from observation table)

Note : If Instrument is not available then fabricate it, using a proper diameter tubes and makes all possible arrangements

Result

Viscosity of given liquid (name of liquid) at room temperature (--°C) was -----------
poise or centipoise (cps), determined by falling ball viscometer (Manufactured by---)

Precautions

1. Viscometer should be cleaned properly and carefully.
2. Put the viscometer on the plane surface through out the experiment so that movement of the ball in the viscometer is uniform and constant
3. First reading should not be recorded because ball can resist more at first instant which gets adjusted properly reducing error due to time.
4. Level in viscometer of both liquid should be similar.
5. Selection of ball depends on the viscosity. Select proper ball for determination of viscosity to minimize error in determination of viscosity.
6. Temperature should be maintained throughout the study by circulating the water in jacket.
7. Take all necessary precautions for the determination of density or specific gravity by pycnometer.

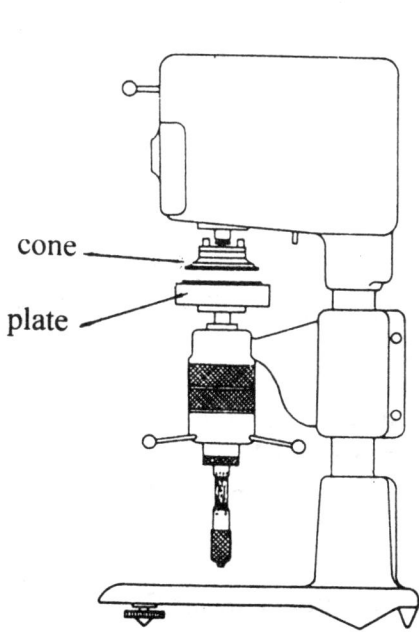

cone

plate

Fig. 4.7. Cone-plate viscometer

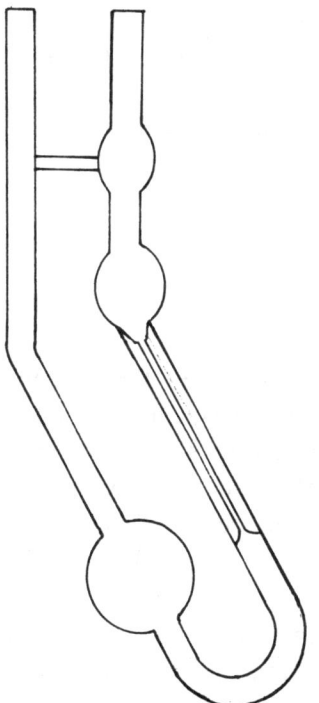

Fig. 4.8. Ostwald- Cannan-Fenske viscometer

EXERCISE NO 4.3

To determine viscosity of liquid using Redwood viscometer

Purpose

- To study the rate of flow of liquid through the orifice.
- To develop concept and handling of Redwood viscometer.

Requirements

Chemicals/reagents

- Glycol
- Or nitrogycerine
- Or simple syrup
- Distilled water
- Washing solution

Equipment /glasswares

- Beaker
- Redwood viscometer
- Pycnometer or Density bottle
- Thermometer
- Balance (Double pan or electronic)
- Stopwatch
- Conical flask
- Measuring cylinder

Procedure

1. Thoroughly clean the viscometer with a mixture of warm chromic acid and if necessary also clean with solvent.
2. After cleaning the viscometer, dry it completely.
3. Rinse the viscometer with purified water, two to three times.
4. Determine the viscosity using pycnometer (as exercise no.3.1).
5. Close the orifice by pinpoint needle and fill 50 ml of purified water in the viscometer cup.
6. Open the orifice and start the stopwatch immediately.
7. Report time taken to pass the 50 ml of purified water through the orifices.
8. Repeat the steps 6 & 7 two to three times.
9. Transfer purified water from the viscometer and rinse with testing liquid two to three times.

10. Fill the 50 ml of testing liquid in the cup of Redwood viscometer as step 5.
11. Open the orifice and start the stopwatch immediately.
12. Report time taken to pass 50 ml of testing liquid through the orifices.
13. Repeat the steps 6 & 7 two to three times.

Observation

(a) Temperature (Room Temperature) =----- °C
(b) Weight of empty pycnometer = -----g
(c) Weight of pycnometer with water = -----g
(d) Weight of pycnometer with testing liquid = -----g

Observation Table

S.No.	Liquid	Time Taken to pass 50 ml of liquid through orifices (sec.)			Average (a+b+c)/3 (sec.)
		I(a)	II(b)	III(c)	
1	Water				
2	Liquid				

Calculation

(a) Calculate density of liquid as given in exercise no. 3.1.
(b) Calculate viscosity of liquid using following formula

$$\eta_1 = \frac{t_1 d_1}{t_2 d_2} \times \eta_2$$

where,
- η_1 viscosity of liquid-----?
- η_2 viscosity of purified water at temperature (--°C).
- d_2 density of purified water at temperature (--°C).
- d_1 density of liquid calculated.
- t_1 Time taken to pass 50 ml of testing liquid through the orifice (taken from observation table).
- t_2 Time taken to pass 50 ml of purified water through the orifice (taken from observation table).

Note : If Instrument is not available then fabricate it using a metallic pipe with curve type bottom having center hole of appropriate radius.

Result

Viscosity of given liquid (name of liquid) at room temperature (--°C) was -----------
poise or centipoise (cps), determined by Redwood viscometer (Manufactured by---)

Precautions

1. Viscometer should be cleaned properly and carefully.
2. Put the viscometer on the plane surface through out the experiment.
3. Orifice must be uniform and should not get affected by solvent.
4. Instrument must be free from rust.
5. Orifice should be clean and free any the obstacle.
6. Accurate and equal volume of purified water and testing liquid should be taken.
7. Orifice must be closed when filling the cup of viscometer so as to avoid leakage.
8. Volume of purified water and testing liquid must be equal in the viscometer.
9. Temperature should be maintained throughout the study by circulatig the water in jacket.
10. Take all precautions necessary for the determination of density or specific gravity by pycnometer.

EXERCISE NO. 4.4

To determine viscosity of paracetamol suspension/shampoo using Ostwald's viscometer

Purpose

- To study the effect of suspending agent in the suspension on viscosity of the final products.
- To study the effect of viscosity on the phamacological response/role of viscosity in the preparation of pharmaceutical product.

Requirements

Chemicals/reagents

- Paracetamol suspension
- Or Shampoo

Equipment /glasswares

Same as exercise no. 4.1

Procedure

1. Prepare paracetamol suspension using given formula or as per the instruction of teacher.
2. Particle of the dispersed phase must be uniform and should not block the capillary of viscometer.
3. Thoroughly clean the viscometer with a mixture of warm chromic acid and if necessary clean with solvent.
4. After cleaning the viscometer, dry it completely by current of hot air or dry in the oven.
5. Shake the suspension properly before filling in the viscometer.
6. Hang the viscometer on the burette stand vertically as shown in the Fig ---------
7. Determine the density of suspension using pycnometer or density bottle (as exercise no. 3.1).
8. Determine the viscosity in the same way as performed in the Ex No-2.1

Observation

(a) Temperature (Room Temperature)   =------°C
(b) Weight of empty pycnometer or density bottle   = -----g
(c) Weight of pycnometer with water   := -----g
(d) Weight of pycnometer with testing liquid   = -----g

Observation Table

S.No.	Liquid	Time Taken to Flow of Liquid between two points(sec.)			Average (a+b+c)/3(sec.)
		I(a)	II(b)	III(c)	
1	Water				
2	Liquid				

Calculation

Calculate density of paracetamol suspension.

Calculate viscosity of liquid using the following formula,

$$\eta_1 = \frac{t_1 d_1}{t_2 d_2} \times \eta_2$$

Where,

- η_1 viscosity of Paracetamol suspension -----?
- η_2 viscosity of purified water at temperature (--°C).
- d_2 density of purified water at temperature (--°C).
- d_1 density of Paracetamol suspension calculated ---?
- t_1 flow time of Paracetamol suspension between two fixed point (taken from observation table)
- t_2 flow time of purified water between two fixed point (taken from observation table)

Result

Viscosity of prepared /given paracetamol suspension at room temperature (--°C) = ------------poise or centipoise (cps), determine by Ostwald viscometer

Precautions

1. Particle size of the suspension should be small so that it can not affect the flow property or can not block the capillary.
2. Flocculated suspension is not suitable for the determination of viscosity using Ostwald viscometer as it gets blocked.
3. All other precautions are same as mentioned in the ex. no. 2.1

Note : Prepare four suspension formulation using different concentration of suspending agent and determine viscosity of all suspensions using same method and plot the graph between concentration of suspending agent and viscosity. It shows increase in viscosity with increase of concentration of suspending agent.

EXERCISE NO 4.5

To determine viscosity of calamine lotion using Redwood viscometer

Purpose

(a) To study the effect of viscosity on application of calamine lotion.
(b) To develop concept and handling of Redwood viscometer.

Requirements

Chemicals/reagents

- Calamine lotion or any suspension

Equipments/glasswares

- Redwood viscometer
- Density bottle

Procedure

1. Prepare calamine lotion by the given formula or as per the instruction the teacher.
2. Reduce the particle size in micron.
3. Thoroughly clean the viscometer with a mixture of warm chromic acid and if necessary cleans the viscometer with solvent.
4. After cleaning the viscometer dry it completely.
5. Rinse the viscometer with purified water two to three times.
6. Shake the calamine lotion before filling in the cup of the viscometer
7. Determine the density of calamine lotion density bottle (as ex. no. 4.3)

Observations

Observation Table

S.No.	Liquid	Time Taken to pass 50 ml through orifices (sec.)			Average (a+b+c)/3(sec.)
		I(a)	II(b)	III(c)	
1	Water				
2	Calamine lotion				

Calculation

Same as exercise no. 4.3

Result

Vscosity of prepared calamine lotion at room temperature (--°C) = -----------poise or centipoise (cps).

EXERCISE NO 4.6

To determine viscosity of liquid paraffin emulsion using falling ball viscometer

Purpose

(a) To study the viscosity of liquid paraffin emulsion.
(b) To develop concept related to the viscosity and its importance in the formulation.

Requirments

Chemicals/reagents

- Liquid paraffin
- Benzoic acid solution
- Vanillin
- Chloroform water

Equipment /glasswares

Same as exercise no. 4.2

Procedure

1. Prepare liquid paraffin emulsion..
2. Reduce the globule size in micron.
3. Same as exercise no. 4.2.
4. Emulsion should be stable and should not show creaming and cracking.

Observation

Observation Table

S.No.	Liquid	Time taken by ball (sec.)			Average (a+b+c)/3(sec.)
		I(a)	II(b)	III(c)	
1	Water				
2	Liquid Paraffin Emulsion				

Calculation

Same as exercise no. 4.2

Result

Viscosity of **prepared liquid paraffin emulsion at room temperature(--°C) =** ------------ poise or centipoise (cps), determined by falling ball viscometer.

EXERCISE NO 4.7

To determine viscosity of shampoo using Ostwald's viscometer

Purpose

- To learn method of determination of viscosity and factor affecting related to consistency.

Requirements

Chemicals/reagents

Same as exercise no. 4.4

Equipments/glasswares

Same as exercise no. 4.4

Procedure

Same as exercise no. 4.4

Observation

Observation Table

S.No	Liquid	Time Taken to flow between two points (sec.)			Average (a+b+c)/3(sec.)
		I(a)	II(b)	III(c)	
1	Water				
2	Shampoo				

Calculation

Same as exercise no. 4.4

Result

Viscosity of prepared Shampoo at room temperature (--°C) was -----------poise or centipoise (cps), determine by falling ball viscometer.

Precautions

1. Prepare shampoo and reduce the separation of layer.
2. Avoid frothing while handling the shampoo.

EXERCISE NO 4.8

To study the effect of temperature on viscosity

Purpose

- To learn the effect of temperature on viscosity.

Requirements

Chemicals/reagents

- Sucrose syrup
- or glycerin & Distilled water

Equipment /glasswares

Same as exercise no. 4.1

Procedure

1. Prepare saturated solution of sucrose in purified water if necessary, filter it without warming the sucrose solution.
2. Arrange the assembly.
3. Before setting the assembly, thoroughly clean the glasswares as well as, equipment required in experiment.
4. After cleaning the viscometer, dry it completely using the current of hot air or dry in the oven.
5. Determine the density of suspension using pycnometer as exercise no. 4.1
6. Report time taken to flow for purified water and sucrose solution under the same conditions between two points, at different temperature.

Observation

(a) Weight of pycnometer or density bottle at room temperature = W_1 g
(b) Weight of pycnometer or density bottle with water represent by = W_w
(c) Weight of pycnometer or density bottle with sucrose solution represent by = W_s

Observation table A

Weight of pycnometer (solutions)	Weight in g					
	Temperature (°C)					
	RT	37	45	55	75	85
W_w W_s						

Observation table B

Liquid	Time Taken to Flow of Liquid between two points (sec.)					
	Temperature (°C)					
	RT	37	45	55	75	85
Water						
Sucrose solution						

Calculation

Calculate density of Sucrose solution at different temperature

$$\eta_1 = \frac{t_1 d_1}{t_2 d_2} \times \eta_2$$

After calculate

Liquid	Density (g/cm^3)					
	Temperature (°C)					
	RT	37	45	55	75	85
Sucrose solution						

Liquid	Viscosity (poise)					
	Temperature (°C)					
	RT	37	45	55	75	85
Sucrose solution						

Result

Viscosity of sucrose solution decreases with increase in temperature. Plot the graph between temperature and viscosity.

EXERCISE NO 4.9

To study the effect of concentration on viscosity

Requirements

Chemicals/reagents

- Sucrose
- or sodium benzoate
- or sodium salicylate

Equipment /glasswares

Same as exercise no. 4.1.

Procedure

1. Prepare different concentration of sucrose solution (5%, 15%, 25%, 35%, 45%, 65%) in purified water at room temperature.
2. Determine viscosity of different concentration of sucrose solution as given in Ex No. 2.1.
3. Determine the density of different concentration of sucrose solution as previous exercise.

Observation

Same as exercise no. 4.1.

Observation table A

Liquid	Weight in g					
	Concentration in (%)					
	5%	15%	25%	35%	45%	65%
W_s						

Observation table B

Liquid	Time taken to flow of liquid between two points (sec.)					
	Concentration in (%)					
	5%	15%	25%	35%	45%	65%
Water Sucrose solution						

Calculation

Calculate density of different concentration of sucrose solution

$$\eta_1 = \frac{t_1 d_1}{t_2 d_2} \times \eta_2$$

After calculation

Liquid	Density (g/cm³)					
	Concentration in (%)					
	5%	15%	25%	35%	45%	65%
Sucrose solution						

Liquid	Viscosity (poise)					
	Concentration in (%)					
	5%	15%	25%	35%	45%	65%
Sucrose solution						

Result

Viscosity of sucrose solution increases with increase in temperature. Plot the graph between concentration of sucrose solution and viscosity

EXERCISE NO 4.10

To prepare different composition of glycerin and water and determine viscosity using Ostwald's viscometer

Purpose

- To study the effect of different composition of glycerin and water on viscosity.

Requirements

Chemicals/reagents

- Glycerin
- Distilled water
- Washing solution

Equipment /glasswares

- Ostwald's viscometer
- Pycnometer or density bottle
- Burette stand
- Balance (Double pan or electronic)
- Stopwatch
- Glassmarker

Procedure

1. Prepare different composition of glycerine and water (20:80. 30:70,40:60, 50:50, 60:40, 70:30) at room temperature.
2. Determine viscosity of different composition of glycerin and water as given in ex no. 4.1.
3. Determine the density of different composition of glycerine and water as ex no. 4.10.

Observation

(a) Temperature (room temperature)   = t°C
(b) Weight of pycnometer or density bottle at room temperature   = W_1 g
(c) Weight of pycnometer + water   = W_w
(d) Weight of pycnometer +different composition of glycerin and water = W_c

Observation table A

Liquid	Weight (g)					
	Composition of glycerin and water					
	20:80	30:70	40:60	50:50	60:40	70:30
W_s						

Observation table B

Liquid	Time taken by liquid to flow between two points (sec.)						
	Composition of glycerine and water						
	0(water)	20:80	30:70	40:60	50:50	60:40	70:30
Composition							

Calculation

Calculate density of different composition of glycerine and water using the formula as given in ex. no. 4.1.

After calculation

Liquid	Density (g/cm^3)					
	Composition of glycerine and water					
	20:80	30:70	40:60	50:50	60:40	70:30
composition						

Liquid	Viscosity(poise)					
	Composition of glycerine and water					
	20:80	30:70	40:60	50:50	60:40	70:30
composition						

Result

Plot the graph between composition of glycerin and water and viscosity.

EXERCISE NO 4.11

To determine composition of unknown mixture of glycerine and water by viscosity

Purpose

- To study the importance of viscosity and its application for the determination of unknown composition of two mixture.

Note – Perfomed as previous exercise no 4.10 and determine the viscosity of the unknown composition in the same way as well as maintain all other standard conditions.

Calculate composition ratio by the graph drawn between the composition of glycerine and water.

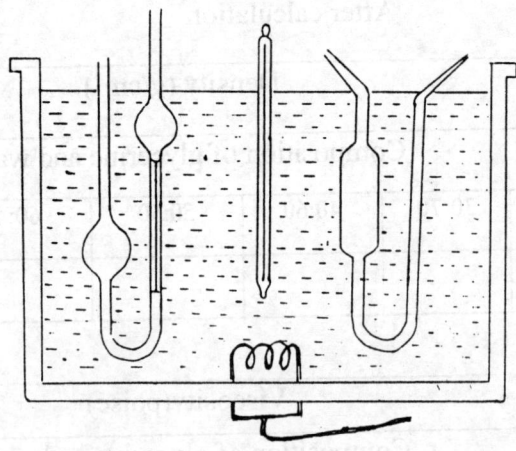

Fig. 4.9. Ostwald's apparatus (laboratory method)

EXERCISE NO 4.12

To determine viscosity of gel using Brookfield viscometer

Purpose

- To learn handling of equipment Brookfield viscometer and determine the viscosity of gels using this instrument because all instrument are not suitable for determination of the viscosity.

Requirements

Chemicals/reagents

- Carbopol-940
- Or sodium alginate
- Or sodium CMC
- Or other gel forming agents
- Distilled water
- Washing solution

Equipment /glasswares

- Brookfield viscometer
- Beaker
- Electric points

Procedure

1. Prepare gel using gel forming agent (Gellant) about 250 g.
2. Put the gel for 24 h for homogenization.
3. Fill the gel in a beaker or gel holder.
4. Select the spindle on the basis of viscosity.
5. Set up the instrument with level of the base and attach with a constant electric supply.
6. Clean the instrument and attach the selected spindle to the viscometer.
7. Rotat the spindle in the gel till get find constant dial reading.
8. Repeat the experiment at least for three times.
9. If you want to study the effect of temperature on viscosity, maintain the temperature for 20 min. and then determine the viscosity.

Observation

(a) Temperature- $= t\ °C$
(b) Amount of gel   = ---- g
(c) Spindle No.   = ------
(d) Speed of the spindle in the gel   = --------
(e) Reading dial average of three readings =

Calculation

Viscosity of the gel= Dial reading × value with the spindle no.& speed (provided by mnufacturer of instrument)

Result

       Viscosity of prepared gel at temperature = --------- poise or centipoise determined by Brookfield viscometer using spindle no-------.

Precaution

1. Prepare homogeneous gel and keep aside for 24 h for homogenization.
2. Take care for selecting proper spindle.
3. Start the instrument at low speed and rotat for least 20 minutes till the dial reading is have constant.
4. After use the instrument is to be clean (cover it or keep in wooden box).
5. Determine the viscosity at constant electric supply as well as constant temperature.

EXERCISE NO 4.13

To determine viscosity of simple ointment using Brookfield viscometer

Purpose

- To learn handling of Brookfield viscometer and determine the viscosity of ointment and compare the result with viscosity of gel.

Requirements

Chemicals/reagents

- Liquid Paraffin
- Hard paraffin
- Soft paraffin
- Lanolin
- Glycerine
- Washing solution

Equipment /glasswares

- Brookfield viscometer
- Beaker
- Electric points

Procedure

1. Prepare simple ointment by the given formula.
2. Perform same as ex. no. 4.12

Observation

(a) Temperature- = °C
(b) Amount of simple ointment = ---- g
(c) Spindle no. = ------
(d) Speed of the spindle in the gel = --------
(e) Dial reading (average of three readings) = ---------

Calculation

Same as exercise no. 4.13.

Result

Viscosity of prepared simple ointment at temperature -------°C = ------oise or centipoise determined by Brookfield viscometer using spindle no-------.

EXERCISE NO 4.14

To study the effect of impurities on viscosity

Purpose

- To learn the effect of impurities on viscosity.

Requirements

Chemicals/reagents

- Sodium chloride/magnesium chloride/Calcium chloride

Equipments/glasswares

Same as exercise no. 4.1

Procedure

1. Prepare, 1%,2%and 3% of sodium chloride, magnesium chloride and calcium chloride solution in purified water.
2. Determine density and viscosity of all solution at room temperature as Ex. No.-2.1

Obsrevations

    (a) Room temperature   =   °C

    (b) Weight of pycnometer (empty and dry)   =   g

Observation table for density

S.No.	Liquid	Weight pycnometer (g)	Flow of liquid			Average (a+b+c)/3 sec.
			a	b	c	
1	purified water					
2	1% NaCl solution					
3	2% NaCl solution					
4	3% NaCl solution					
5	1% MgCl$_2$ solution					
6	2% MgCl$_2$solution					
7	3% MgCl$_2$solution					
8	1% CaCl$_2$solution					
9	2% CaCl$_2$ solution					
10	3% CaCl$_2$ solution					

Calculation

Determine viscosity and density of different solution using the formulal as given in ex. no.-4.1.

Result

Viscosity of liquids increases with increasing of impurities in the liquids. Plot the bar diagram between liquid and viscosity obtained by experimental dala.

EXERCISE NO 4.15

To study the effect of polarity on viscosity (ethanol, glycol and glycerol)

Purpose

- To study the effect of polarity on the viscosity.
- To learn the effect of hydrogen bonding on the viscosity.

Requirements

Chemicals/reagents

- Ethanol (C_2H_5OH)
- Glycol (HO-CH_2-CH_2-OH)
- Glycerol (HO-CH_2- CH(OH)- CH_2-OH)

Equipment /glasswares

Same as exercise no. 4.1

Procedure

1. Determine density and viscosity of ethanol, glycol, and glycerol liquids at room temperature as ex. no. 4.1.

Observations

Same as exercise no. 4.1

Observation Table for density

S.No.	Liquid	Weight (g)	Flow of liquid			Average (a+b+c)/3 sec.
			A	b	c	
1	Purified water					
2	Ethanol					
3	Glycol					
4	Glycerol					

Calculation

Determine viscosity and density of different solution using the formula as given in ex.no. 4.1.

Result

Viscosity of liquids increases with increase in of hydrogen bonding.
Plot the bar graph between liquid and viscosity obtained by experimental dala..

Viva-voce Question Bank

1. What is viscosity?
2. Why viscosity is determine?
3. How to determine the viscosity of liquids?
4. Give factors affecting flow of liquids.
5. Define flow properties of liquids.
6. What is dilatant flow?
7. How to determine the pseudoplastic flow of liquid?
8. Give principle of Ostwald viscometer.
9. How to measured viscosity of liquid by Ostwald viscometer?
10. What is plug flow? Explain with examples.
11. What is yied value?
12. Explain Newtonian and Non-Newtonian flow of liquid.
13. What is the role of thixotropy in the formulation?
14. Give advantages and disadvantages of Ostwald viscometer.
15. Explain mobility and fluidity with examples.
16. Describe working principle of Brookfield viscometer.
17. Describe the rheological behaviour of syrups, suspension, emulsion and semi solids.
18. Give principle of Redwood viscometer?
19. Define kinematic viscosity with examples.
20. How to determine the viscosity of gels?
21. What is the criteria for selection of the viscometers.
22. How to measure viscosity by the falling sphere viscometer.
23. Explain viscoelasticity with suitable examples.
24. Define psychorheology with examples.
25. What is the main role of viscosity in the manufacturing of pharmaceutical products.

❑❑❑

Chapter 5

SURFACE TENSION

The area adjacent to two phases is called as interface or interfacial region. In pharmacy, various heterogeneous dosage forms are commonly used, viz.

* Suspension (solid dispersion in the liquid medium or continuous phase)
* Emulsions (two immiscible liquids like oil and water)
* Powder (solid in vapor, powder in contact with body surface)

Classification of Interfaces

Interfaces are mainly divided in following categories

Phases in contact	Example
Gas in Gas	No interface possible
Gas in liquid	Aerosol, Carbonated water
Gas in solid	Solid surface in contact with air (gas)
Liquid in liquid	Two immiscible liquids, benzene and water, cyclohexane and water
Liquid in solid	Dispersion of solid in liquid
Solid in solid	Powder particles in contact with body surface

Surface Tension

In a bulk portion of phase, molecules are attracted by other molecules equally in all directions. The surface phase is also in a state of tension because the molecules present on the surface are constantly acted upon by three forces in the direction perpendicular to each another and out of which two forces are equal and opposite and hence cancel each other. The remaining force acting on the surface molecules causes tension on the surface which is called as surface tension .The molecule inside the phase of liquids is free of this force because it has equal and opposite forces in all direction (Fig. 5.1). Hence surface tension can be defined as 'the force in dynes acting on a surface at right angles to any line of unit length.'

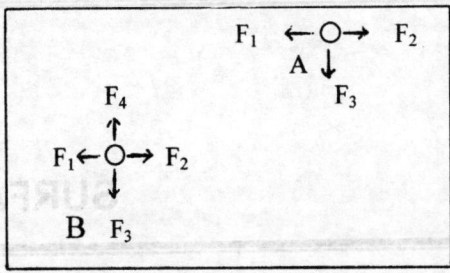

Fig. 5.1. Representation of unequal attractive forces on molecules

Force on molecule B is

$$F_B = F_1 + (-) F_2 + F_3 + (-)F_4 \qquad\qquad -- (5.1)$$

where, $F_1 = F_2$, and $F_3 = F_4$ are equal and opposite forces

Hence,

$$F_B = 0$$

Force on molecule A is

$$F_A = F_1 + (-) F_2 + F_3$$

where, $F_1 = F_2$, is equal and opposite forces

Hence,

$$\boxed{F_A = F_3 \text{ (surface tension)}} \qquad\qquad --- (5.2)$$

As defined, surface tension of the liquid can be determined by the following equation

$$\boxed{\text{Surface tension } (\gamma) = \frac{F}{L}} \qquad\qquad --- (5.3)$$

where, γ is a Greek symbol represents the surface tension, F is force perpendicular to the length L.

Unit of surface tension is Newton/meter or N/m in M.K.S. and dynes/cm in C.G.S. system.

The presence of tension on the interfaces can be explained by the following experiment. Take circular metallic frame, a looped piece of thread loosely tied in the frame. Dip the frame in soap solution to form a film. When it is removed from the soap solution and exposed to the air, a film of liquid will be stretched entirely across the circular frame. If the liquid inside the loop is punctured or removed by a warm pin carefully, the loop will be converted into a stretched circular shape as shown in Fig. 3.2.

Another example for presentation of surface tension is-, Consider three-sided wire frame which has a movable bar. A soap film is formed inside the frame and than stretched by applying a force to the movable bar. Here length of the bar works against the surface tension of the soap film. Hence the surface tension of solution forming the film is the function of the film that applied to break the film with the length of the movable bar.

$$\text{Surface tension} = \frac{\text{Force applied on the bar to break the film}}{\text{Length of the movable bar}}$$

$$\text{Surface tension } (\gamma) = \frac{F}{2l} \qquad \text{--- (5.4)}$$

2l is the length of the movable bar because the soap film has two interfaces liquid in gas, one above and one below the plane of the paper.

Surface Free Energy

Surface tension maintains the minimum surface area of liquids. Hence surface free energy is equal to work required to increase the $1 cm^2$ area of a liquid. According to Fig. 3.3 surface free energy calculated by the following equation-

$$\text{Work} = \text{force} \times \text{displacement of bar from AD to A'D'}$$

$$W = F \times d \qquad \text{-- (5.5)}$$

Substitute value of F by equation from the equation (5.4)

$$W = \gamma \times 2l \times d \qquad \text{--- (5.6)}$$

If surface area of bar $\Delta A = 2l \times d$

Hence equation (5.6) is

$$\boxed{W = \gamma \times \Delta A} \qquad \text{--- (5.7)}$$

Interfacial Tension

Interfacial tension is the force per unit layer working at the interfaces between two immiscible liquid phases. Interfacial tension is always less than surface tension because the adhesive forces between two liquid phases forming an interface are greater than when a liquid and a gas phase exist together.

Factors Affecting Surface Tension

1. Temperature
2. Concentration
3. Hydrogen bonding
4. Surface active agents
5. Suspending agent
6. Polarity
7. Impurities
8. Other factors

Methods for Measurement of Surface Tension and Interfacial Tension

Many methods are employed for the measurement of surface tension and interfacial tension such as

1. Capillary rise method
   a. Single capillary rise method
   b. Double capillary rise method
2. Drop fall method
   a. Drop weight mehtod
   b. Drop number method
3. DuNouy tensiometer method
4. Bubble pressure method
5. Sessile drop method
6. Wilhelmy plate method

Three methods are generally employed for the determination of surface tension and interfacial tension in the laboratory. viz. Drop number, capillary rise, and DuNouy ring method .These methods are discussed here.

Drop number method

This is the simplest method for the determination of surface tension of liquid in the laboratory. The method is based on the principle that a fixed volume (weight of liquid W) of the liquid is delivered as freely falling from a capillary tube held vertically, it is approximately proportional to the surface tension of the liquid.

Surface tension $\propto$ weight

$$\gamma \propto W \qquad \text{--- (5.8)}$$
$$\gamma = \frac{F}{2l} \qquad [F = mg]$$

Circumference of the drop = $2\pi r$, it is equal to the length of the bar
Hence equation is presented in this form
$$2\pi r\, \gamma = mg = V\rho g$$
If V, volume contains n drops, than weight of one tablet is
$$2\pi r\, \gamma = mg\, /n = V\rho g/n$$
$$2\pi r\, \gamma = V\rho g/n$$
$$\gamma = V\rho g\, /\, 2\pi r n \qquad \text{--- (5.9)}$$

If densities of two liquids ρ_1 and ρ_2, the number of drops of two liquids be n_1 and n_2 for the same volume V of the liquids from two fixed points respectively. Applying equation (5.10) and determine the surface tension of liquid while the radius of tube is same.

$$\gamma_1 = V\rho_1 g\, /\, 2\pi \qquad \text{-- (5.10)}$$
$$\gamma_2 = V\rho_1 g\, /\, 2\pi r n_1 \qquad \text{--- (5.11)}$$

Equation (5.10) is divided by Equation (5.11)
$$\frac{\gamma_1}{\gamma_2} = \frac{V\rho_1 g\, /\, 2\pi r n_1}{V\rho_2 g\, /\, 2\pi r n_2} = \frac{\rho_1\, /\, n_2}{\rho_2\, /\, n_2}$$

$$\boxed{\frac{\gamma_1}{\gamma_2} = \frac{\rho_1\, n_2}{\rho_2\, n_1}} \qquad \text{--- (5.12)}$$

If the surface tension of one liquid is known then the surface tension of other liquids is calculated by the equation-5.12. n_1 and n_2 determined by the counting drops of both liquids using *Traube stalagmometer* (Fig. 5.2) and density of liquids can be determined by the pycnometer or density bottle as discussed in chapter 2.

Capillary rise method

When a capillary is dipped into a liquid in a beaker, it is observed that liquid generally rises up till a certain height. It is due to higher force of adhesion between the liquid molecules and the capillary wall than the cohesion between the liquid molecules wetting the wall of the capillary and results in rising of liquid in capillary. The height of liquid is dependent on the type of liquids and wetting power to the tube. Using this principle, it is possible to measure the surface tension of liquid but using this method interfacial tension of liquids can not be determined. Suppose a liquid of density ρ rises in a capillary tube inside radius r and height of liquid rises in the tube is h (Fig. 5.3), then two forces are working in the capillary tube.

(a) Force (F_1) due to surface tension, raising the liquid column upward

F_1 = inside circumference of capillary × surface tension of liquid

$F_1 = 2\pi r\gamma$

(b) Force (F_2) of gravity pulling the liquid downward

F_2 = weight of liquid in the column pulled downward due to gravity

$F_2 = mg$

if, $m = \rho V$ and V (volume of liquid inside the tube) = $\pi r^2 \times h$

Hence,

$$F_2 = \pi r^2 \times h\rho g = \pi r^2 . h\rho g$$

At the equilibrium state both forces are equal

$$F_1 = F_2$$

or $$2\pi r\gamma = \pi r^2 \times h\rho g$$

or $$\boxed{\gamma = \tfrac{1}{2}\, rh\rho g}$$ -- (5.12)

If the liquid has poor wetting power or wetting is not pertect, in this condition contact angle (θ) between glass and liquid is not zero.

Hence,

$$F_1 = 2\pi r\gamma \cos\theta$$

Now equation (5.12) is

$$\boxed{\gamma = rh\rho g / 2\cos\theta}$$ --- (5.13)

DuNouy Tensiometer

DuNouy tensiometer is commonly used for determination of surface tension and interfacial tensions. It is very convenient, rapid and require small amount of sample. The principle of the instrument depends on the fact that the force required to detach a platinum-iridium ring immersed at the surface or interface is proportional to the surface tension or interfacial tension. The force which is necessary to dettach the ring in this manner that is provided by a torsion wire and is recorded in dynes on a calibration dial. The instrument is shown in the Fig. 5.4. The surface tension of liquid is determined by the following equation.

$$\gamma = \frac{\text{Dial reading in dynes}}{2 \times \text{ring circumference}} \times \text{correction factor}$$

EXERCISE NO. 5.1

To determine surface tension of liquid using stalagmometer.

Purpose

- To learn concepts of surface tension and its utility.

Requirements

Chemicals/reagents
- Distilled water
- Ethyl acetate
- or benzene
- or nitrobenzene
- or toluene
- or carbon tetrachloride

Equipments/glasswares

- Pycnometer
- Thermometer
- Beaker 100 ml, and 250ml
- Burette stand
- Weight box
- Weighing balance

Procedure

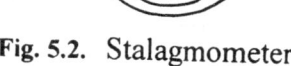

Fig. 5.2. Stalagmometer

1. Thoroughly clean the pycnometer and stalagmometer using chromic acid and purified water or as because surface tension is highly affected with grease or other lubricants
2. Stalagmometer must be mounted in the vertical plane using burette stand.
3. Fill the purified water in the instrument and count the number of drops falling down between two points of the instrument as shown in Fig. 5.2.
4. Repeat the step-3 at least three times.
5. Rinse the stalagmometer using the same liquid of which surface tension is to be determined.
6. Fill the stalagmometer by liquids and count the number of drops formed between two points as step 3.epeat the steps 6 at least three times for accuracy.
7. Density of the liquid is determined using pycknometer as given in experiment 2.2 at the same temperature.

Observations

(a) Temperature (room temperature) $= t\,°C$
(b) Weight of empty pycnometer $= w_1$
(c) Weight of pycnometer + distilled water $= w_2$
(d) Weight of pycnometer + liquid $= w_3$

Observation table

Liquid	Number of drops				Specific gravity	Surface tension
	(i)	(ii)	(iii)	Mean		
Water				$n_1 =$		
Liquid				$n_2 =$		

Calculation

(a) Weight of liquid $= w_3 - w_1$
(b) Weight of distilled water $= w_2 - w_1$
(c) Specific gravity of liquid $(\rho_2/\rho_1) = (w_3 - w_1)/(w_2 - w_1)$

$$\gamma_2 = \frac{\rho_2\, n_1}{\rho_1\, n_2} \times \gamma_1$$

Calculate the surace tension of liquid by this equation, γ_1 is the surface tension of water obtain from the table (appendix)

Result

Surface tension of given liquid at room temperature $(t\,°C)$ = -------- dynes/cm.

EXERCISE NO. 5.2

To determine surface tension of liquid using capillary rise method.

Purpose

- To learn concept of surface tension and its application in the field of pharmacy.

Requirements

Chemicals/Reagents

- Distilled water
- Liquid

Equipments/Glasswares

- Pycnometer
- Thermometer
- Beaker 100 ml, 250ml and 1 L.
- Burette stand
- Capillary tube
- Microscope
- Weighing balance

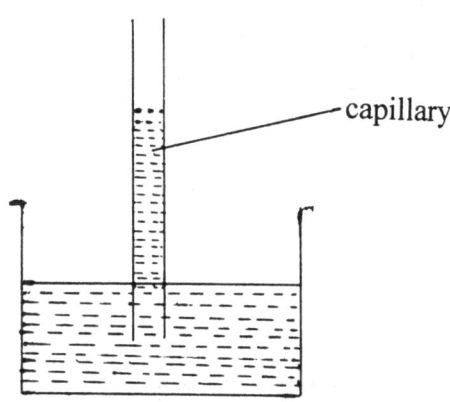

Fig. 5.3. Diagram capillary tube

Procedure

1. Clean the capillary tube using solvent and dry it.
2. Take test liquid in the beaker.
3. Dip the capillary in the liquid vertically.
4. Liquid will rise in the capillary & after some time, obtain a maximum height in the capillary.
5. Record liquid level initially in the beaker and maximum level rise in the capillary by cathetometer.
6. Density of the liquid is determined by the pycnometer as exercise no. 3.1.
7. Radius of the capillary is measured by the microscope.

Observation

(a) Temperature (room temperature) $= t\ °C$
(b) Weight of empty pycnometer $= w_1\ g$
(c) Weight of pycnometer + distilled water $= w_2\ g$

(d) Weight of pycnometer + liquid   = w_3 g
(e) Initial reading of the cathetometer   = h_1 cm
(f) Final reading of the cathetometer   = h_2 cm
(g) (Maximum liquid level in the capillary)
(h) Least count of eye-piece (oculometer)   = ----μm
(i) Diameter of the capillary   = d cm

Calculation

(a) Weight of liquid   = $w_3 - w_1$
(b) Weight of distilled water   = $w_2 - w_1$
(c) Specific gravity of liquid $(\rho_2/\rho_1) = (w_3 - w_1)/(w_2 - w_1)$
(d) Density of liquid $(\rho) = (w_3 - w_1)/(w_2 - w_1) \times 1$

Surface tension of liquid is determined by the following equation

$$\gamma = r\,h\,\rho\,g\,/\,2$$

where ρ is the density of liquid

Result

The surface tension of liquid at t °C = ---------------dynes/cm.

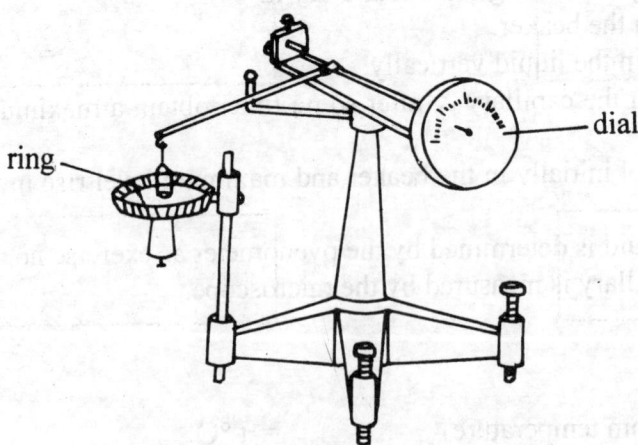

Fig. 5.4. Conco DuNouy tensiometer

EXERCISE NO 5.3

To determine surface tension of liquid using DuNouy tensiometer.

Purpose

- To learn the principle and handling of DuNouy tensiometer for determination of the surface tension.

Requirements

Chemicals/reagents

- Ethyl alcohol
- Purified water

Equipments/glasswares

- Tortion balance
- Platinum ring
- Thermometer

Procedure

1. Clean the apparatus with hot acid and rinse it using distilled water.
2. Heat the platinum wire to redness in a luminous flame.
3. Hang this wire on the beam without touching it.
4. Turn the knob until the pointer reach at zero and adjust the torsion of the wire by the screw so that beam lies on the horizontal position.
5. Put a small piece of paper on the ring and twist the wire until the beam is reached at horizontal position.
6. Record the reading of the pointer on the scale.
7. Place weight 50, 100, 150, and 200 mg one by one and record the torsion angle.
8. Plot a graph between the weight and torsion angle. It will be linear shows the torsion of wire is proportional to the torsion angles.
9. Remove the piece of paper and weights and set the beam in horizontal position at zero reading of the scale.
10. Take small amount of test liquid in a clean watch glass on the platform.
11. Raise the platform by the help of lift screw until the liquid just touches the ring.
12. The beam will tilt towardsdown side due to the surface

Observation

(a) Temperature (room temperature) = t °C
(b) Radius of the ring = R cm
(c) Weight of the paper piece = w_1 g

Observation table for calibration

S.No.	Weight of the ring (mg)	Torsion head reading in deg. (B)	Weight force in g (A)	Torsion angle in g (y = B / A)
1.	Paper			
2.	50			
3.	100			
4.	150			
5.	200			

Observation table for surface tension of liquid

S.No.	Liquid	Torsion head reading (x)	Weight force in g (m = x / y)	Torsion angle in (γ = mg / 4 π R)
	Water			
	Liquid			

Calculation

Calculate weight force F from the pointer reading and the calibration curve and then determine the surface tension of liquid and mixture of liquid.

Result

The surface tension of liquid = ------ dynes / cm.

EXERCISE NO. 5.4

To determine parachor of the given liquid by surface tension method using stalagmometer.

Purpose

- To learn the method of determination of parachor.
- To learn the utility of parachor in the pharmaceutical science.

Requirements

Chemicals/reagents

- Ethyl alcohol
- Methyl alcohol
- Benzene
- Purified water

Equipments/glasswares

- Pycnometer
- Stalagmometer
- Beaker 100 ml, 250ml and 1 L.
- Burette stand

Procedure

1. Determine density of each liquid at room temperature as in exercise no 5.1.
2. Clean the stalagmometer using soap solution and rinse it two to three times with distilled water, if necessary, rinse it acetone or ether.
3. Fill the water in stalagmometer and count the number of drops between two point as exercise no. 5.1.
4. Remove the water and rinse with the same liquid to be used for the determination of surface tension.
5. Fill the liquid and count the number of drops between two point as consider for water.
6. Repeat the experiment at least three time and use its mean for calculation.

Observations

(a) Temperature (room temperature) $= t\ °C$
(b) Weight of empty pycnometer $= w_1$
(c) Weight of pycnometer +distilled water $= w_2$

(d) Weight of pycnometer +methyl alcohol   = w_3
(e) Weight of pycnometer +ethyl alcohol   = w_4
(f) Weight of pycnometer +benzene   = w_5

Observation table

S.No.	Liquid	Number of drops (i)	(ii)	(iii)	Average number of drops	Surface tension (dynes / cm)	Parachor of liquid
1.	Water						
2.	Methy alcohol						
3.	Ethyl alcohol						
4.	Benzene						

Calculations

(A) Calculate density of liquids

Same as exercise no. 5.1

(B) Calculate surface tension of liquids

Same as exercise no. 5.1 using the following formula

$$\gamma_2 = (n_1\rho_2) / (n_2\rho_1) \times \gamma_1$$

Where γ_1 surface tension of liquid and ρ_1 & ρ_2 densities of water and liquid res pectively.

(C) Calculate parachor of liquids

Parachor of the liquids is determined using following equation

$$P = \frac{\text{Molecualar weight of liquid} \times (\text{surface tension of liquid})^{1/4}}{\text{density of liquid}}$$

Result

Parachor of the given liquids =----, ---- and -------.

EXERCISE NO. 5.5

To determine surface tension of benzene and n-hexane using stalagmometer

Purpose

- To learn the effect of pi-bond in the compound on surface tension.
- To study the surface tension of cyclic compound and their property.

Requirments

Chemicals/reagents
- Benzene
- Cyclohexane
- Purified water

Equipments/glasswares
- Stalagmometer
- Pycnometer
- Thermometer
- Beaker 100 ml, 250ml and 1 L.
- Burette stand

Procedure

1. Clean the stalagmometer by detergent solution and with distilled water and finally rinse with acetone.
2. Arrange stalagmometer in the burette stand and place on the plane surface.
3. Dip the mouth of the stalagmometer in water and suck the distilled water carefully and avoid air bubble and sputum inside the apparatus.
4. After a fix point start counting of the drops till another point as shown in Fig. 5.2.
5. Take other reading and perform same as exercise no. 5.1
6. Take at least three reading of each sample.
7. Determine density of liquid as in exercise no.3.2.
8. Calculate the surface tension.

Observations

    (a) Temperature (room temperature) $= t\,°C$
    (b) Weight of empty pycnometer $= w_1$
    (c) Weight of pycnometer + distilled water $= w_2$
    (d) Weight of pycnometer + benzene $= w_3$
    (e) Weight of pycnometer + cyclobenzene $= w_4$

Observation table

S.No	Liquid	Number of drops			Average number of drops	Surface tension (dynes / cm)
		(i)	(ii)	(iii)		
1.	Water					
2.	Benzene					
3.	Cyclohexane					

Calculations

(A) Calculate density of liquids

Same as exercise no. 5.1

(B) Calculate surface tension of liquids

Same as exercise no. 5.1 using the following formula

$$\gamma_2 = (n_1\rho_2) / (n_2\rho_1) \times \gamma_1$$

Where γ_1 surface tension of liquid and ρ_1 & ρ_2 densities of water and liquid respectively.

Result

The surface tension of given liquids = ------- dynes / cm and ------- dynes / cm.

EXERCISE NO. 5.6

To study the effect of temperature on surface tension

Purpose

- To learn the effect of temperature on the surface tension.

Requirements

Chemicals / reagents

- Carbon tetrachloride
- Purified water

Equipments/glasswares

- Stalagmometer
- Pycnometer
- Thermometer
- Water bath or beaker of 1L

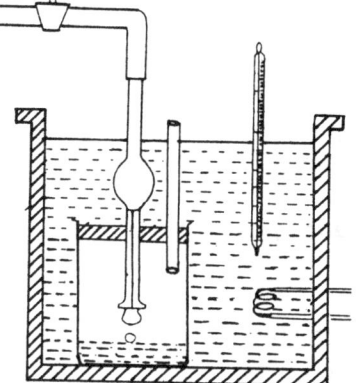

Fig. 5.5. Stalagmometer

Procedure

Same as exercise no. 5.1

Observations

Temp. (°C)	Number of drops			Average number of drops	Number of drops			Average number of drops	Surface tension (dynes / cm)
	(i)	(ii)	(iii)		(i)	(ii)	(iii)		
RT									
37									
45									
55									
65									
75									

Calculation

Same as exercise no. 5.3.

Result

Plot the graph between temperature and surface tension of liquid so that result can be obtained in the form of increasing or decreasing order.

EXERCISE NO 5.7

To study the effect of concentration on surface tension

Purpose

To learn concepts of density and its utility

Requirments

Chemicals/reagents

- Sodium benzoate
- Sodium salicylate
- or liquid
- Purified water

Equipments/glasswares

- Stalagmometer
- Pycnometer
- Thermometer
- Burette stand
- Weight box
- Weighing balance

Procedure

1. To prepare different concentration of the sodium salicylate or sodium benzoate (0.1%, 0.2%,-------9.0% and 1.05) or different dilution of the liquid.
2. Clean the apparatus of stalagmometer by cleaning solution and if necessary with the solvent.
3. Dip the stalagmometer in the distilled water and suck it carefully.
4. Start counting of drops between two point as shown in the fig.----
5. The velocity of the water should be controlled by attaching a clip with the rubber tube.
6. Take at least three reading.
7. Remove water and clean the stalagmometer and the apparatus rinse & it with acetone .
8. Similarly fill the liquid in stalagmometer and start the counting in the same way.
9. Take reading of all sample.
10. Record the number of drops in table form and calculat surface tension of liquid at different concentration.
11. Plot the graph between concentration and surface tension.

Observation

1. Temperature (room temperature) $= t \, °C$
2. Weight of empty pycnometer $= w_1$
3. Weight of pycnometer + distilled water $= w_2$
4. Weight of pycnometer + benzene $= w_3$
5. Weight of pycnometer + cyclobenzene $= w_4$

Observation table

S.No.	Concentration	Number of drops			Average number of drops	Surface tension (dynes / cm)
		(i)	(ii)	(iii)		
1.	Water					
2.	Sodium bezoate 0.1%					
3.	0.2%					
4.	0.3%					
5.	0.4%					
6.	0.5%					
7.	0.6%					
8.	0.7%					
9.	0.8%					
10.	0.9%					
11.	1.0%					

Calculations

Same as exercise no. 5.1 using the following formula

$$\gamma_2 = (n_1 \rho_2) / (n_2 \rho_1) \times \gamma_1$$

Result

The surface tension of given liquid at different concentration = -----and ---dynes / cm
Plot the graph between concentration and surface tension and respect the effect of concentration on surface tension.

EXERCISE NO. 5.8

To prepare different composition of glycerin and water and determine surface tension using stalagmometer.

Purpose

- To learn the effect of dilution on the surface tension.
- To study the effect of concentration on surface tension.

Rrequirements

Chemicals/reagents

- Glycerin

Equipments/glasswares

Same as exercise no. 5.5

Procedure

Same as exercise no. 5.5

Observation table

S.No.	Concentration	Number of drops			Average number of drops	Surface tension (dynes / cm)
		(i)	(ii)	(iii)		
1.	Water					
2.	Glycerin1.0%					
3.	2.0%					
4.	3.0%					
5.	4.0%					
6.	5.0%					
7.	6.0%					
8.	7.0%					
9.	8.0%					
10.	9.0%					
11.	10.0%					

Calculations

Same as exercise no. 5.1.

Result

The surface tension of given liquid at different composition of glycerin and water = -----and ---dynes/cm. Plot the graph between different composition of glycerin and water and surface tension and report the result on the basis of graph.

EXERCISE NO 5.9

To determine composition of liquids by surface tension

Purpose

- To learn method of determination of unknow concentration of the given composition of liquid by surface tension method.

Requirements

Chemicals/reagents
- Glycerin
- Purified water

Equipments/glasswares

Same as exercise no 5.8

Procedure

Same as exercise no. 5.8

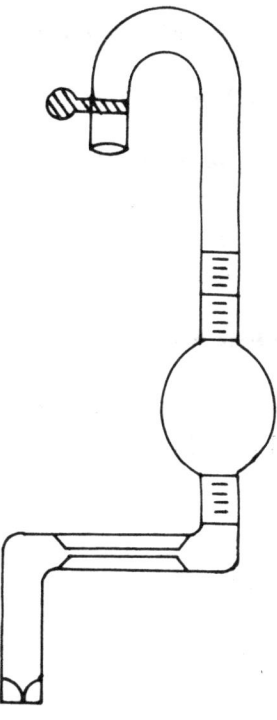

Calculations

Same as exercise no. 5.1

$$\gamma_2 = (n_1\rho_2) / (n_2\rho_1) \times \gamma_1$$

Fig. 5.6. Stalagmometer

Result

Plot the graph between different composition of glycerin & water and surface tension. Determine surface tension of unknown sample by the graph.

The concentration of the unknown sample = --- %.

EXERCISE NO. 5.10

To study the effect of surfactant on surface tension.

Purpose

- To learn the effect of surfactant on the surface tension.

Requirements

Chemicals/reagents

- Detergent & Surfactant

Equipments/glasswares
Same as exercise no. 5.1

Procedure
Same as exercise no. 5.1

Observation

Same as exercise no. 5.1

Procedure

Observation table

S.No.	Concentration of surfactant	Number of drops			Average number of drops	Density (g/cm^3)
		(i)	(ii)	(iii)		
1.	Water					
2.	Surfactant 0.2%					
3.	0.4%					
4.	0.60%					
5.	0.8%					
6.	1.0%					
7.	1.2%					
8.	1.4%					
9.	1.6%					
10.	1.8%					
11.	2.0%					

Calculations
Same as exercise no. 5.1

Result

The surface tension of the liquid increases/decreases with the increasing the concentration of surfactant.

EXERCISE NO. 5.11

To study the effect of impurities on surface tension.

Purpose

To learn effect of impurities on density and its utility

Requirements

Chemicals/reagents

- Sodium chloride/Calcium chloride/Magnesium chloride

Equipments / glasswares

Same as exercise no. 5.1

Procedure

Observation table

S.No.	Concentration of salt	Number of drops			Average number of drops	Density (g/cm³)
		(i)	(ii)	(iii)		
1.	Water					
2.	Salt 0.2%					
3.	0.4%					
4.	0.60%					
5.	0.8%					
6.	1.0%					
7.	1.2%					
8.	1.4%					
9.	1.6%					
10.	1.8%					
11.	2.0%					

Calculations

Same as exercise no. 5.1

$$\gamma_2 = (n_1 \rho_2) / (n_2 \rho_1) \times \gamma_1$$

Result

Plot the graph between different concentration surfactant of and surface tension. The surface tension of the liquid increases/decreases with increase in the concentration of surfactant.

EXERCISE NO. 5.12

To study the effect of polarity on surface tension.(ethanol and glycol)

Purpose

- To learn the effect polarity on surface tension.

Requirments

Chemicals / reagents

- Ethanol/glycol/glycerol

Equipments/glasswares

Same as exercise no. 5.5

Procedure

1. Temperature (room temperature) $= t\ °C$
2. Weight of empty pycnometer $= w_1$
3. Weight of pycnometer + distilled water $= w_2$
4. Weight of pycnometer + Ethanol $= w_3$
5. Weight of pycnometer + glycol $= w_4$
6. Weight of pycnometer + glycerin $= w_5$

Observation table

S.No.	Liquid	Number of drops			Average number of drops	Density (g/cm^3)
		(i)	(ii)	(iii)		
1.	Water					
2.	Ethyl alcohol					
3.	Glycol					
4.	Glycerin					

Calculations

Same as exercise no. 5.1

$$\gamma_2 = (n_1\rho_2) / (n_2\rho_1) \times \gamma_1$$

Result

Plot the graph between different liquids and surface tension. The surface tension of the liquid increase/decrease with the increasing the polarity of the liquids.

Viva-voce Question Bank

(A) Short answer type question
1. What is surface tension?
2. What is the effect of temperature on surface tension?
3. How to measure surface tension in the laboratory?
4. Give principle of drop weight method for determination of surface tension.
5. What is the difference between surface tension and parachor?
6. What is the difference between surface tension and interfacial tension?
7. What is surface free energy?
8. Give factors affecting the surface tension.
9. Define interfaces with examples.
10. Give classification of interfaces.
11. Explain mechanism of capillary method.
12. Justify that drop number method is better than drop weight method.
13. Draw labelled diagram of stalagmometer.
14. Define surfactant and its application.
15. What is spreading coefficient?
16. Why you determine surface tension?
17. How to increase surface tension?
18. How to decrease surface tension?
19. Why surface tension of benzene is greater than the alkanes of comparable molecular weight?
20. Explain surface tension and interfacial tension with atleast one example.in each case.

(B) State true/false

1. Surface tension is expression in units of dynes/cm^2.
2. Surface free energy is expressed in units of eargs/ cm^2.
3. The work required to create a unit area of surface, known as the surface free energy per unit area equivalent to the surface tension of a liquid system.
4. The force per unit radius of interface generally is called as the interfacial tension.
5. Surface free energy $W = \gamma \Delta P$.
6. Surface tension of water decreases with increase in of temperature.
7. Surface tension of glycerine is less than water.
8. Surface tension of water at 20°C is 72.8 dynes/cm.
9. DuNouy tensiometer is widely used to measure surface tension and not suitable to measure interfacial tension.
10. $\gamma = 1/2r\rho hg$

Answer (B) State true/false
1. F 2. T 3. T 4. F 5. F 6. T 7. T 8. T 9. F 10. T

Chapter 6

SOLUBILITY

Solubility is an important phenomenon in pharmaceutical sciences. It plays very effective and prominent role in the formulations of dosage forms. Solubility of a compound in a particular solvent is defined as the concentration of the solute (compound) in a saturated solution at a certain temperature. In another term, it may be defined as the continuous interaction of two or more compound to form homogenous molecular dispersion. On the basis of solute and solvent present in the solution, it can be classified in three categories.

Saturated solution

Saturated solution is one in which the substance (solute) is in equilibrium with the solid phase at a particular temperature. In these types of solution, the solute is completely in the soluble state.

Unsaturated solution

It is a solution which containing the less amount of solute than the saturated solution at a particular temperature.

Supersaturated solution

A supersaturated solution is one that contains more substance than required for the preparation of the saturated solution at a definite temperature. Solubility of the solute is enhanced by changing the physical parameters.

Solubility may be expressed in a concise form by J.W.Gibb. It is useful for relating the effect of variables on solubility like temperature, pressure, concentration etc. upon the various phases such as solid, liquid and gaseous.

$$F = C - P + 2$$

--- (6.1)

where F is degree of freedom in the system, C is the number of components and P represents the number of bases. This equation is known as Gibb's phase rule or equation.

$$ice \leftrightarrow water \leftrightarrow vapor$$

In this example component (C) = 1 and number of phases (P) = 3

Expression of solubility

Many terms are used for the expression of solubility. When quantitative data are available, solubility may be expressed in many ways like molarity, molality, normality, formality, mole fraction, and percent solution. In pharmaceutical sciences, solubility can be expressed in the following terms.
(a) % w/w (weight by weight) (b) % w/v (weight by volume)
(c) % v/v (volume by volume)

Solubility of the drugs is expressed in various units in the Merck Index.

Table 6.1. Terms used for solubility

Term	Parts of solvent required for 1 part of solute
Very soluble	Less than 1 part
Freely soluble	1 to 10 parts
Soluble	10 to 30 parts
Sparingly soluble	30 to 100 parts
Slightly soluble	100 to 1000 parts
Very slightly soluble	1000 to 10,000 parts
Practically insoluble	More than 10,000 parts

Factors Affecting Solubility

Many factors are affecting solubility of substances in solvents viz.
• Temperature
• Concentration
• Types of solute & types of solvent
• pH
• Particle size
• Molecular structure
• Common ion effect
• Combined effect of solvent and pH
• Effect of complex formation
• Effect of wetting agent or surfactant
• Effect of non-electrolytes

Determination of Heat of Solution by Solubility Method

Heat of solution is measured by Van't Hoff equation at two different temperatures by the following equation

$$\frac{d \log S}{dT} = \frac{\Delta H}{RT^2}$$ --- (6.2)

where, S is the solubility of the solute in solvent, ΔH is the heat of solution and T is the absolute temperature. It is considered that the heat of solution is dependant on the temperature, hence the equation 4.5 written as

$$\int_{S1}^{S2} d \log S = \Delta H / R \int_{T1}^{T2} 1 / T^2 \, dt$$ --- (6.3)

$$\log_e S_2 - \log_e S_1 = \Delta H / R(1 / T_1 - 1 / T_2)$$ --- (6.4)

$$\log_{10} S_2 - \log_{10} S_1 = \Delta H / 2.303R(1 / T_1 - 1 / T_2)$$ --- (6.5)

If solubilities S_1 and S_2 of substance at two different temperature

Determination of Solubility

For determination of solubility of a solid in liquids, it can be divided into two steps

1. Preparation of saturated solution

Saturated solution of substance can be prepared by three methods. All three methods are employed for the preparation of saturated solution in practice but second method is more preferable than the first and third methods because this method is fast and easy to prepare the saturated solution.

(a) In first method, the substance is added in the solvent slowly at a particular temperature and solute is not added more than the saturation.

(b) The second method is based on the effect of temperature, as solubility increases with increase in temperature. If the solubility is to be studied at 25°C, then the solvent is to be heated at 30° to 35°C with excess amount of solute. The amount of solute required is more at higher temperature for the preparation of saturated solution. When this solution is cooled at the study temperature (25°C) the excess amount of solute is separated out in the solution. It can be separated by the filtration. The filtrate solution is considered as saturated solution at the study temperature.

(c) The third method is same as second method but is slightly different from the second, as in this method excess amount of the solute is added in solvent at the study temperature and shaken with continuous stirring or by wrist action shaker for few hours or left the container for 24 h for saturation. With occational shaking and removing excess amount of solute by filtration. This solution is known as saturated solution.

2. Analysis of saturated solution

The analysis of saturated solution depends on the nature of the substance (solute) and accuracy of analysis. Many methods have been employed for the determination of solubility.

(a) *Evaporation method*

This method is suitable for those substances which do not decompose at a slightly higher (10-20°C) temperature than the boiling point of a solvent. In this method a suitable volume of the saturated solution of the solute in solvent at the study temperature is weighed in a porcelain dish and the solvent is evaporated till dryness. It is heated to achieve a final volume in an oven to a constant weight. Thus, the amount of the solid present in the solution can be calculated.

(b) *Volumetric method*

This method is suitable for determination of solubility of acids and bases by titration. In this method a fixed volume of solution is treated with a suitable reagent using an indicator and determine amount of the solute present in the solution. This method is suitable for the determination of solubility in the solvent.·

(c) *Gravimetric method*

This method is suitable to those substances which react with reagents in solution and gives sparingly soluble product. In this method, a known quantity of solution is taken and added suitable reagent to precipitate the substance completely into the form of new compounds or salt form. Filtrate the precipitate and remove the solvent if necessary wash the precipitate using purified water and then dry the precipitate. Weighed amount of precipitate is to be drird in the porcelin dish to get a constant weight. By this method solubility can be calculated as the number of grams of solute in 100 g of the solvent.

(d) *Instrumental methods*

All these methods are very sensitive and suitable for determination of solubility in fractions or in micron. Instrumental methods are very popular for the determination of solubility due to its ease of working and simplicity.

(a) UV-spectrophotometer method
(b) High Performance Liquid Chromatography (HPLC)
(c) Thin Layer Chromatography (TLC)
(d) Gas Chromatography (GC)
(e) Many other methods

EXERCISE NO. 6.1

To determine the solubility of an inorganic salt at different temperature.

Purpose

- To study the parameters of solubility and to have understanding of familiar with saturated solution.
- To learn method of preparation of saturated solution and its importance.

Requirements

Chemicals/reagents

- Pure inorganic salts (KCl, NaCl, NaNO$_3$, K$_2$SO$_4$ etc.)
- Distilled water

Equipments/Glasswares

- Thermostat
- Thermometer
- Porcelain dishes or watch glasses
- Beaker (50 ml,100 ml, and 250 ml)
- Pipette (10 ml)
- Hot plate

Procedure

1. Clean all glasswares using detergent solution and chromic acid solution.
2. Wash two to three times using purified water.
3. Take 50 ml of distilled water in a beaker (100 ml).
4. Add some amount of salt like potassium chloride or sodium chloride in distilled water and stir using glass rod or by an electric motor driven shaker.
5. Increase the temperature to 85°C with contineous stirring.
6. Maintain this temperature for few minutes and then cool down the solution.
7. Take sample at 80°C using a pipette with a piece of filter paper, tie at the tip of the pipette so that the insoluble salt can be removed.
8. Remove the piece of filter paper from the tip of pipette and transfer 10 ml of this solution in weighed porcelain dish or watch glass.
9. Allow the temperature to fall down slowly to 70°, 60°, 50°, 40,° 30°C and then to room temperature.
10. At each temperature take sample of the solution and repeat the step 7 and step 8.
11. Evaporate the solution of each porcelin dish or watch glass using direct heat or on

the water bath or put in the oven.

12. Dry the solution till constant weight.

13. Take weight of the dish using double pan balance or chemical balance and calculate weight of the powder.

14. Record all the parameter in the form of table or in proper way so that it becomes easy to understand the concept of solubility.

Observations

Observation table

S. N.	Tempe-rature (°C)	Weight of empty Dish w_1 g	Weight of dish + solution w_2 g	Weight of dish + residue w_3 g	Weight of residue $w_3 - w_1$ g	Weight of solvent $w_2 - w_3$ g	Solubility in g /100 g
1	80						
2	70						
3	60						
4	50						
5	40						
6	30						
7	RT						
8	20						
9	10						
10	5						

Calculations

Solubility of salt in solvent at temperature (°C) is calculated by the following formula in g /100 g.

$$\text{Solubility of salt at 80°C} = \frac{w_3 - w_1}{w_2 - w_3} \times 100$$

Result

Solubility of the given salt at room temperature (considering the saturated solution at room temperature) = ------ %. Plot the graph between solubility and temperature. The graph will show a smooth curve without any break.

Note : Solubility of the salt can be determined below the room temperature using cold water in the thermostat.

EXERCISE NO. 6.2

To determine the solubility of benzoic acid at room temperature and below the room temperature (10°C) by volumetric method.

Purpose

- To learn determination of solubility by titration using phenolphthalein as an indicator (acid base balance).
- To study the effect of temperature on solubility of benzoic acid.

Requirements

Chemicals/reagents

- Benzoic acid
- Sodium hydroxide
- Hydrochloric acid
- Phenolphthalein indicator
- Distilled water

Equipments / Glasswares

- Thermostat
- Thermometer
- Conical flask
- Beaker (50 ml,100 ml, and 250 ml)
- Pipette (10 ml)

Procedure

1. Thoroughly clean all glasswares using detergent and chromic acid solution.
2. Rinse the glassware two to three times using distilled water and dry completely in the oven.
3. Take 25 ml of distilled water in a beaker and heat slightly at more than room temperature and add excess amount of benzoic acid in the beaker with constant stirring.
4. Cool this beaker at room temperature.
5. Take 5 ml of supernatant liquid from the saturated solution at room temperature and transfer in a conical flask.
6. Titrate this solution using standardized 0.1N NaOH and phenolphthalein as an indicator.

7.Repeat step 5 and step 6 at least three times.

8.In another flask take 25 ml of distilled water in a beaker and cool it at 10°C.

9.Add excess amount of benzoic acid and repeat step 3 to step 6.

10.All datas presented in the form of table.

Observations

(a) Indicator for titration phenolphthalein

(b) Equivalent weight of benzoic acid   = 122

(c) Normality of prepared NaOH   = ----- N

(d) Sample withdrawn at both temperature   = 5 ml

(e) Solubility study at room temperature or any other temperature = --- °C

Observation table A

S.N.	Temperature (°C)	Burette reading		Volume of 0.1N NaOH required for neutralization (b – a) ml
		Initial reading (a)	Final reading (b)	
1				
2	Room Temp.			
3				

Observation table B

S.N.	Temperature (°C)	Burette reading		Volume of 0.1N NaOH required for neutralization (b – a) ml
		Initial reading (a)	Final reading (b)	
1				
2	10			
3				

Calculation

A. Calculation of solubility of benzoic acid at room temperature (--- °C)

Normality of benzoic acid

$$N_1V_1 = N_2V_2$$
$$\text{solution} \qquad \text{alkali}$$

or

$$N_1 = N_2V_2 / V_1 \qquad\qquad \text{--- (6.6)}$$

where, N_1 is normality of solution, V_1 is the volume of solution withdrawn at room temperature for titration, N_2 is the normality of NaOH and V_2 is the volume required of NaOH required to neutralize the withdrawn solution. Calculate N_1 using the equation 6.6.

Solubility of Benzoic acid at room temperature is determined by the following formula
Solubility of benzoic acid per 100 ml of solution (M)

$$M = \frac{N_1 E \times 100}{1000} \text{ g / 100 ml}$$ --- (6.7)

B. Calculation of solubility of benzoic acid at room temperature (--- °C)

Normality of benzoic acid –

$$N_3 V_3 = N_2 V_2$$
solution   alkali

or $$N_3 = N_2 V_2 / V_3$$ --- (6.8)

where, N_3 is normality of solution at 10°C , V_3 is the volume of solution withdrawn at 10°C for titration, N_2 is the normality of NaOH and V_2 is the volume required of NaOH required to neutralize the withdrawn solution. Calculate N_3 using the equation 4.3.
Solubility of Benzoic acid at 10°C is determined by the following formula
Solubility of benzoic acid per 100 ml of solution (M)

$$M = \frac{N_3 E \times 100}{1000} \text{ g / 100 ml}$$ --- (6.9)

Result

Solubility of benzoic acid at room temperature (---°C) is ----%, while solubility at 10 °C is ----%.

Precautions

1. All glassware should be clean and dry .
2. While transferring the solution from the pipette to volumetric flask, only supernatant liquid should be taken.
3. Standardize the sodium hydroxide solution using phenolphthalein indicator.
4. Repeat the titration three times till you obtain equal volume for Neutralization of the solution.
5. The pipette should be warmed by sucking hot water two to three times if you want to determine the solubility at more than the room temperature.
6. For determination of solubility at 10°C, the pipette should be kept at the same temperature by circulation of cool water three to four times.
7. End point of the titration should be determined carefully.
8. Calculate concentration of benzoic acid at different temperature.

EXERCISE NO. 6.3

To determine the heat of solution of substance by solubility method

Purpose

To learn the method for determination of heat of solution

Requirements

Chemicals/Reagents

- Benzoic acid
- Distilled water

Equipments / Glasswares

Same as exercise no. 6.1

Procedure & Observations

Same as exercise no. 6.1

Calculation

Solubility of benzoic acid is determined at two different temperature T_1 and T_2 while solubilities S_1 and S_2 respectively. The heat of the solution is determined by the following equation

$$\log_{10} S_2 - \log_{10} S_1 = \Delta H / 2.303R(1 / T_1 - 1 / T_2)$$

where ΔH is heat of solution

Result

The heat of solution of oxalic acid = ------ cals. / mole.

Note : In place of oxalic acid take any acid like benzoic acid etc or other materials for this exercise

EXERCISE NO. 6.4

To study the effect of additive of an electrolyte on the solubility of an organic acid at room temperature

Purpose

- To learn the effect of electrolytes on the solubility of an acid

Requirements

Chemicals/reagents

- Benzoic acid
- Potassium chloride
- or sodium chloride
- or sodium sulphate

Equipments / glasswares

Same as exercise no. 6.1

Procedure

1. Prepare saturated solution of benzoic acid slightly higher temperature then the room temperature about to 250 ml.
2. Cool the solution at room temperature.
3. Remove the undissolved material by filtering the saturated solution of the benzoic acid.
4. Take this solution 30 ml in 5 flask and place the proper level on the container.
5. Add 1, 2, 3, 4, and 5 g of potassium chloride in the respective container.
6. Shake the flask for 2 min. and left for 10 minutes for the settling of the undissolved material.
7. Filter this solution in another labeled container.
8. Determine the solubility of the benzoic acid without electrolyte (potassium chloride) by titration with 0.05 M sodium hydroxide using phenolphthaline as indicator.
9. Repeat the experiment at least three times.
10. Determine the solubility of the benzoic acid in the different solution in the same way as above by 0.05 M sodium hydroxide.
11. Plot the graph between concentration of the electrolytes and solubility of the acid and report the result.

Observations

   (a) Temperature (room temperature) $= t\ °C$

   (b) Indicator for titration Phenolphthalein

   (c) Normality (molarity) of sodium hydroxide $= 0.05\ M$

   (d) Electrolytes use potassium chloride

Observation table

S.No.	Amount potassium chloride added (g)	Volume of solution containing KCl (ml)	Burette reading		Volume of 0.05 M NaOH used	Solubility (%)
			Initial reading	Final reading		
1.	Blank	10				
		10				
2.	1	10				
		10				
3.	2	10				
		10				
4.	3	10				
		10				
5.	4	10				
		10				
6.	5	10				
		10				

Calculation

Calculate the solubility of the acid per 100 g of the solvent by acid base titration as exercise no. 6.1.

Result

Plot the graph between the solubility and concentration of the potassium chloride and report the result.

Note : In this exercise it may be possible to prepare different concentration of the potassium chloride solution and excess quantity of the benzoic acid and determine the solubility of the benzoic acid.

EXERCISE NO. 6.5

To study the effect of temperature on solubility of paracetamol

Purpose

- To learn the effect of temperature on the solubilty of poorly water soluble drug

Requirements

Chemicals/reagents

- Paracetamol
- Distilled water

Equipments/glasswares

- UV-visible spectrophotometer
- Thermostat
- Dissolution apparatus
- Stirrer

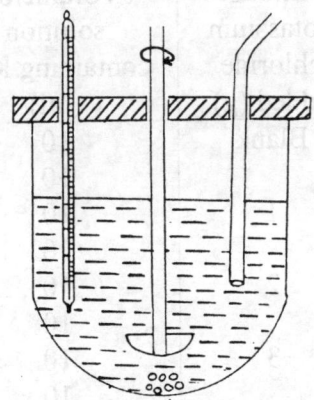

Fig. 6.1. Dissolution apparatus

Procedure

1. Clean the dissolution apparatus (in place of this apparatus take 500 ml beaker and used stirrer and put this beaker on hot plate or on the hot plate magnetic stirrer)
2. Take about to 250 ml of distilled water in the container.
3. Add excess amount of paracetamol.
4. Increase the temperature with constant stirring and take 10 ml of the sample.
5. After each sample add 10 ml of distilled water.
6. Prepare standard curve of paracetamol using distilled water as blank
7. Measure the absorption by spectrophotometer or titration at different temperature
8. Determine solubility of drug.
9. Plot the graph between temperature and solubility of the paracetamol in distilled water

Observations

Observation table

S.No.	Temperature (°C)	Volume of sample taken	Absorbance	Concentration of paracetamol (µg /ml)
1.	RT			
2.	37			
3.	45			
4.	65			
5.	75			
6.	85			
7.	95			
8.	105			
9.	115			
10.	125			

Calculation

Calculate the amount of drug dissolved at different temperature in µg /ml

Result

Plot the graph between temperature and concentration of the drug dissolved at different temperature. Solubility of the paracetamol increases/decreases with the increase of temperature.

Note : Take any sample in place of paracetamol which is slightly soluble in the distilled water or any buffer solution. Solubility can be also be calculated at different pH using buffer solution.

EXERCISE NO. 6.6

To study the effect of stirring on solubility of paracetamol

Purpose

- To learn the effect of stirring on solubility

Requirements

Chemicals/reagents

Same as exercise no. 6.5

Equipments/glasswares

Same as exercise no. 6.5

Procedure

1. Arrange the instrument as in exercise no. 6.5
2. Add excess amount of the drug.
3. Perform other steps same as in exercise no. 6.5 except increase the temperature, change speed of the stirrer at room temperature or any constant temperature.
4. Determine the amount of drug in μg / ml.
5. Plot the graph between speed of stirring and concentration of the drug.

Observations

Observation table

S.No.	Speed of stirrer (rpm)	Volume of sample taken	Absorbance	Concentration of paracetamol (μg /ml)
1.	50			
2.	100			
3.	150			
4.	200			
5.	250			

Calculation

Calculate the amount of drug dissolved at different temperature in μg /ml

Result

Plot the graph between speed of stirrer and concentration of the drug dissolved at room temperature. Solubility of the paracetamol increases/decreases with the increase in speed of stirrer.

EXERCISE NO. 6.7

To study the effect of particle size on solubility

Purpose

- To learn the effect of particle size on the solubility of the drug

Requirements

Chemicals/reagents

- Paracetamol or any other substances
- Buffer solution
- Distilled water

Equipments/glasswares

- Different sieves (30, 45, 60, 80, 100, 140, and 200)
- Dissolution apparatus
- Other glasswares
- Sieve shaker
- Thermometer

Procedure

1. Sieves are arranged in a nest with the coarsest at the top.
2. Place this sieve set on a mechanical shaker apparatus.
3. Shake the powdered drug for a period of 10 min.
4. Collect material from the different sieve size.
5. Take weighed amount of uniform size of the powdered material and measure the concentration of drug at constant pH, constant stirring rate and maintain uniform temperature.
6. Solubility of the drug is determined by the spectrophotometry.
7. The absorbance of the drug should be noted carefully or if necessary dilute the sample according to the range of the standard curve of the drug.
8. In place of drug take some other chemicals or drug also as per the availability of the material.
9. Take precaution for the estimation of the sample.

Observations

(a) Temperature (room temperature) = t °C
(b) pH of the medium = ------
(c) Speed of the stirrer = 50 rpm

Observation table

S.No.	Material retained on the sieve no.	Volume of sample taken	Absorbance	Concentration of paracetamol (µg /ml)
1.	30			
2.	45			
3.	60			
4.	80			
5.	100			
6.	140			
7.	200			

Calculation

Calculate the amount of drug dissolved in distilled water or other medium, obtained from the different sieve in µg /ml

Result

Plot the graph between particle size of powder (sieve size powder retained on the sieve) and concentration of the drug dissolve at room temperature. Solubility of the paracetamol increases/decreases with the decreasing of the particle size.

EXERCISE NO. 6.8

To study the effect of solubilizing agent on solubilization

Purpose

- To learn the effect of solubilizing agent on the solubility of poorly soluble drug in the distilled water.

Requirements

Chemicals/reagents

- Sodium benzoate
- Sodium salicylate
- Polyethylene glycol
- Urea
- Ascorbic acid
- Paracetamol or other poorly soluble drug in the water

Equipments/glasswares

Same as in exercise no. 6.6

Procedure

1. Prepare solution of different concentration of solubilizing agent in water (1%, 2%, 3%, 5%, etc.)
2. If any undissolved material in the solution, filter it.
3. Add excess amount of drug in each solution and shake it at constant temperature and constant speed of the stirrer.
4. Take sample after a fix interval of time or stir the solution at a fix time 15 min. and measured amount of drug dissolved by spectrophotometer or by the titration of the sample.
5. At the same condition take another sample of the solubilizing agent and measure the solubility of the material.
6. By this exercise, one can study two effect at a time, first is the effect of concentration of the solubilizuing agent and second to found out which material dissolved more drug /material at particular condition.
7. Optimize the solubility parameter by considering all factors affecting solubility.

Observations

(a) Temperature (room temperature) = t °C
(b) pH of the medium = ------
(c) Speed of the stirrer = 50 rpm

Observation table

S.No.	Concentration of solubilizing agents (%)	Volume of sample taken	Absorbance	Concentration of paracetamol (µg /ml)
1.	Sod.benzoate 1%			
2.	2%			
3.	3%			
4.	4%			
5.	5%			
6.	PEG 1%			
7.	2%			
8.	3%			
9.	Urea 1%			
10.	2%			
11.	3%			
12.	4%			
13.	5%			

Calculation

Calculate the amount of drug dissolved in distilled water containing different concentration of the solubilizing agent.

Result

Plot the graph between different concentration of the solubilizing agent and concentration of the drug dissolved at room temperature. Solubility of the paracetamol increases/decreases with the increase in solubilizing agent ---------.

Viva-voce Question Bank

(A) Short answer type question
 1. What is solubility?
 2. Why are you studying solubility?
 3. How to determine solubility?
 4. What is solution?
 5. Classify solution with examples?
 6. What is difference between solution and solubility?
 7. What is cosolvency?
 8. What is micellar solubilization?
 9. How to determine the solubility of a solid in liquid?
10. How to determine the solubility of a liquid in liquid?
11. What is the effect of particle size on solubility?
12. What are the precautions to be taken while determining the solubility of a substance?
13. Give factors affecting the solubility of gas in liquid.
14. Give factors affecting the solubility of liquid in liquid.
15. Give method of expression of solubility.
16. What is the role of solubility in the preparation of dosage forms?
17. How to enhance the solubility of gas in liquid?
18. How to reduced the solubility of gas in liquid?
19. What is common ion effect?
20. How to determine generation of heat by solubility?

(B) State true / false
 1. Substances used as solubilizing agents have HLB value less than 5.
 2. Chloramphenicol is poorly soluble in water.
 3. Aspirin is highly soluble in water.
 4. The solubility of poorly soluble substances is enhanced by use of more than one solvent. This phenomenon is known as cosolubilization.
 5. Generally solubility increases with decrease in particle size.
 6. Henry's law is generally applied on solubilisation of solid in liquid.
 7. Crystalline solids have high solubility.
 8. The effect of pressure on the solubility of a gas is expressed by Gibb's law.
 9. Bunsen coefficient is defined as the volume of gas in liters that dissolves in 1 liter of solvent.
10. PEG is used as solubilizing agents.

Answer (B) State true / false
         1. F   2. T   3. F   4. T   5. T   6. F   7.F   8. F   9. T   10. T

❑❑❑

Chapter 7

VAPOR PRESSURE

Both solid and liquid posses a vapor pressure which is a measure of the tendency of the substance to evaporate. There is a certain pressure on the liquid due to its vapor. The magnitude of pressure depends on the temperature and types of liquid. If a liquid is closed in an evacuated container, there would be molecule of the substance in the vapor state over the liquid and they exert a definite pressure on the liquid.

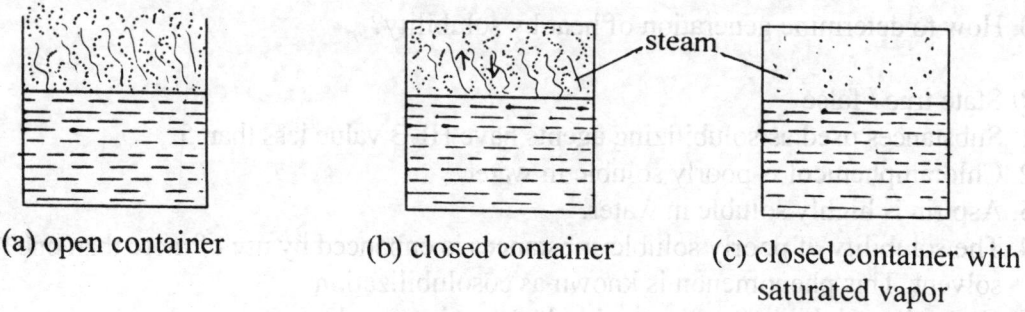

(a) open container   (b) closed container   (c) closed container with saturated vapor

Fig. 7.1. Representation of vapor pressure

The molecules continually leave the surface and reach into the free space, some molecules return to the surface of the liquid (Fig.7.1. a) depending on their concentration in the vapor. After some times a condition of equilibrium is reached (Fig.7.1.b) where the rate of escape equals to the rate of return.

At equilibrium

Rate of vaporization of molecules $\rightleftharpoons$ Rate of condensation of molecules

The pressure of vapor, which exists over any liquid or solid at any temperature, the equilibrium position having been attained, is called *vapor pressure*. When the vapor is in equilibrium with its liquid, it is said to be saturated vapor, when the vapor is less than this value, the vapor is called as unsaturated. Vapor pressure of liquid depends on the temperature, but not on the quantity of liquids. If the values of the vapor pressure plotted against temperature it exhibits curve as follows.

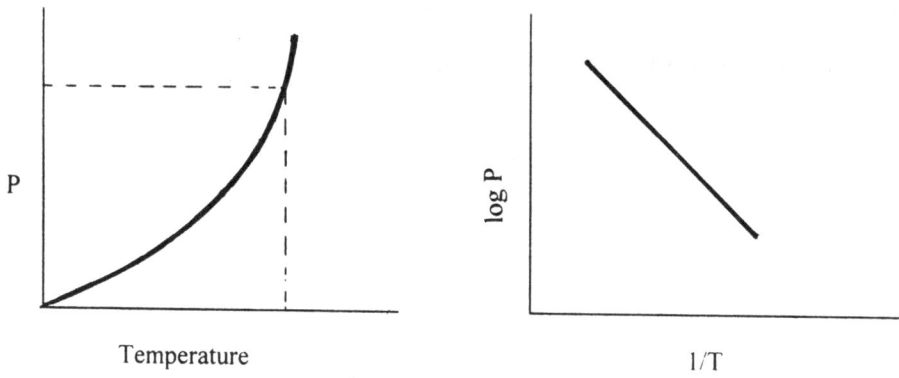

Fig. 7.2. Model of vapor pressure-temperature curve

In this process heat is absorbed and, therefore, the vapor pressure increases with temperature. As the temperature is increased further, the density of the vapor raised and that of the liquid decreases. After all, the densities equal to each other and liquid and vapor can not be distinguished. The temperature at which this take place is called the critical temperature and above it there can be no liquid phase.

When the vapor pressure of a liquid is equal to the pressure applied externally, the liquid boils and evaporated freely. At 100°C, the vapor pressure of water is 760 mm and hence water boil at 100°C.

Factors Affecting Vapor Pressure

- Temperature
- Polarity of substances
- Hydrogen bonding
- Molecular weight

Vapor pressure of a liquid is raised with temperature at which its value is equal to atmospheric pressure is known as the boiling point of the liquid. The quantitative dependence of boiling point upon pressure can be determined by the use of the Clapeyron-Clausius equation, which may be expressed as

$$\frac{dp}{dt} = \frac{\Delta H_v}{T\,(V - V_l)} \qquad \text{--- (7.1)}$$

where, ΔH_v is the molecular latent heat, V_1 and V are volumes of liquid and vapor respectively at the absolute temperature T. dp/dT is the rate of change of vapor pressure with temperature is dependent upon the latent heat.

If $V >>>> V_1$

$$\frac{dp}{dT} = \frac{\Delta H_v}{T\,V}$$

It can be assumed that the vapor obeys the gas laws,

Hence, $\qquad PV = RT \qquad$ or $\quad V = RT/P$

$\therefore \qquad\qquad \dfrac{dp}{dT} = \dfrac{\Delta H_v P}{RT^2}$

Solve this equation

$$\frac{1.\,dp}{P.\,dT} = \frac{d \log p}{dT}$$

Hence,

$$\frac{d \log p}{dT} = \frac{\Delta H_v}{RT^2}$$

After integration of this equation with the limit of pressure p_1 to p_2 and temperature limit is T_1 and T_2, we get

$$\log_{10}\frac{p_2}{p_1} = \frac{2.303\,\Delta H_v}{R} \left[\frac{1}{T_1} - \frac{1}{T_2}\right]$$

where, p_1 and p_2 are the vapor pressure at absolute temperature of T_1 and T_2 respectively and R is a constant, which is equal to 1.987 calories.

Determination of Vapor Pressure

Two methods are commonly employed for measuring the vapor pressure of liquids

1. Static method

In this method a liquid is evaporated in Torricellian vacuum and depression of the mercury column is noted at a specific temperature. The maximum variation in mercury column is equal to the vapor pressure of the liquid evaporated. Vapor pressure may be determined with a suitable manometer or a differential manometer is attached to improve the accuracy of measurement. Some devices are used for the determination of vapor pressure such as

(a) *Smit and Menzier Devices*

This is a convenient static method for the direct measurement of the vapor pressure. This instrument is also known as *isoteniscope* (Fig. 7.3). The liquid is half filled into the small bald A and the liquid stands about half-way up the limbs of the U-tube B. The whole assembly is immersed in a constant temperature bath and a pressure gauge and large bottle are connected at C. Air of the apparatus is removed and pressure is reduced until the liquid in bulb A begins to boil. The pressure is adjusted until the level of liquid becomes same in both limbs of B. The pressure shown by the manometer is the vapor pressure of the liquid at the specific temperature.

(b) *Ramsey and Yound devics*

This method is used to obtain results of a high degree of accuracy. The apparatus consists of a boiling tube with strong walls. The apparatus is shown in Fig. 7.5. It consists of the following parts
    (a) boiling tube
    (b) Pressure gauge consists of a long tube dipping into mercury
    (c) Large bottle
    (d) Tube attached to a capillary
    (e) Tape

2. Dynamic method

In this method the liquid is made to boil under a definite pressure at specific temperature. The external pressure is equal to the vapor pressure of the liquid at this temperature.

EXERCISE NO. 7.1

To determine vapor pressure of pure water at different temperature

Purpose

- To study the effect of temperature on vapor pressure
- To learn about vapor pressure determination methods and its accuracy

Requirements

Chemicals/reagents

- Distilled water

Equipments/glasswares

- Beaker two 100 ml and 250 ml
- Conical flask
- Thermometer
- Glass rod
- Mercury
- Vacuum pump
- Smith and Menzies apparatus

Procedure

1. Arrange the assembly as shows in the Fig.7.3.
2. Fill the bulb B about to two third with purified water and place in the tube A containing paraffin oil and attached the bulb B to the thermometer.
3. Check the apparatus for any types of leakage.
4. Admit some air through D and increase the temperature of the bath to 30°C, stir the bath liquid well and maintain the constant temperature.
5. Reduce the pressure by opening the stopcock and then connect it to the exhaust pump.
6. Falls of pressure first due to air bubbles and later due to bubbies of vapor arising from the bulb B because of the boiling of the liquid under reduced pressure.
7. Close the cork F and allow the liquid to boil continuously till all air bubble is removed completely from the bulb.
8. Temperature of this assembly is noted by the thermometer.
9. The vapor pressure of the liquid at recorded temperature is determined by the manometer reading.
10. Recorded vapor pressure of water at different temperature.

Observations

Barometer reading (atmospheric pressure) = P_1 mm. Hg

Observation table

Temperature (°C)	Manometer reading P_2 mm.Hg	Vapor pressure $(P_1 - P_2)$ mm.Hg
25		
35		
45		
55		
65		
75		
85		

Calculations

Calculate the value log p and plotted the graph between log p and 1/ T. It will show a straight line which can be represented by the following expression,

$$\log p = A - B/T$$

Determine the temperature at which the vapor pressure of the water is p = 760 mm, by extrapolating the graph.

Result

The vapor pressure of water at --------- and - °C are -----------and – mm respectively.

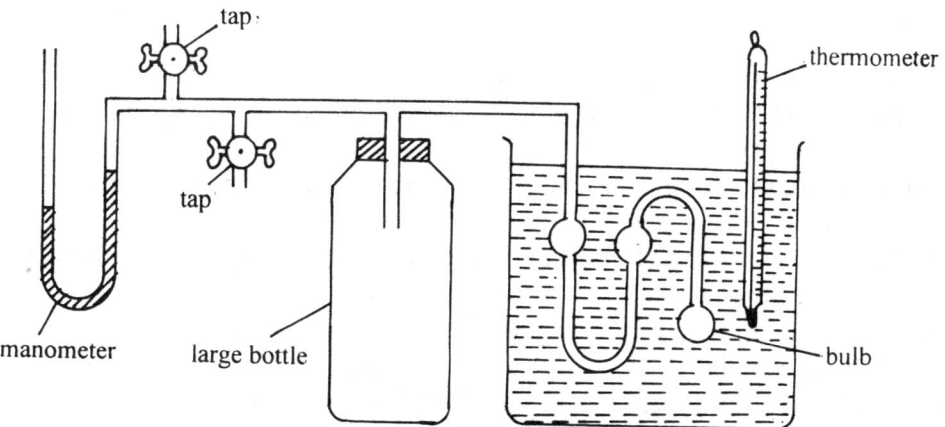

Fig. 7.3. Smith and Menzies apparatus

EXERCISE NO. 7.2

To determine the vapor pressure of benzene at different temperature

Purpose

- To learn the effect of temperature on the vapor pressure and study its importance.

Requirements

Chemicals/reagents

- Benzene
- Mercury
- Distilled water
- Paraffin oil
- Other substances

Equipments/glasswares

- Beaker
- Conical flask
- Distillation assembly
- Thermometer
- Manometer
- Vacuum pump or suction pump

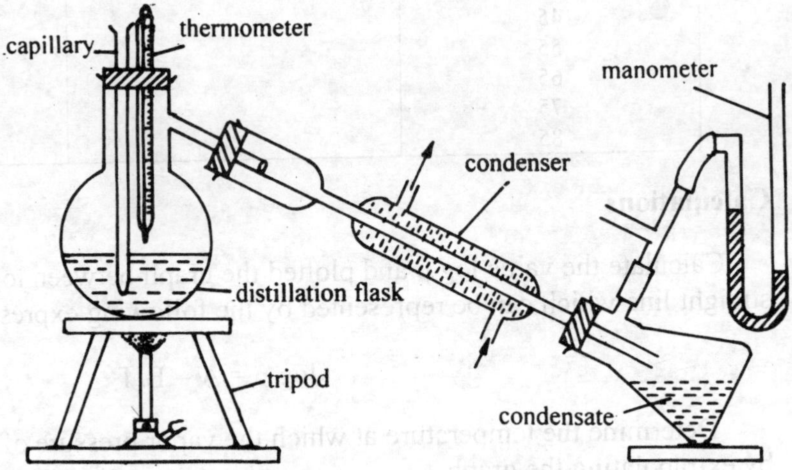

Fig. 7.4. Distillation apparatus

Procedure

1. Arrange the apparatus as shown in the Fig.7.4.
2. Fill about 150-200 ml of benzene in the round bottom flask A and fit a thermometer and a fine capillary.*
3. Keep the valve closed and evacuate the system as fast as possible till the boiling of the liquid starts.
4. Stop the evacuation and slightly open the valve and enter some air into the system and then close the valve.
5. Slowly heat the liquid until the liquid starts boiling and start distillation at the rate of about 1 drop/seconds.
6. Record the temperature and reading of manometer.
7. Increase the temperature slightly by opening the valve.
8. Further heat the liquid so that it just boils continuously distills over. Record the temperature using thermometer and reading of manometer.

9. Repeat the step 7 and 8.
10. Similarly record the temperature and manometer reading and determine the boiling point at different pressures.
11. Finally report pressure by barometer.

Observations

Barometer reading (atmospheric pressure) = P_1 mm. Hg

Observation table

Temperature (°C)	Manometer reading P_2 mm.Hg	Vapor pressure $(P_1 - P_2)$ mm.Hg

Calculations

The difference of barometer pressure and the pressure difference of the manometer give the vapor pressure of the liquid at equilibrium temperature. Calculate the value log p and plotted the graph between log p and 1/ T. It will show a straight line and which can be represented by the following expression,

$$\log p = A - B/T$$

Determine the temperature at which the vapor pressure of the liquid p = 760 mm, by extrapolating the graph.

Result

The vapor pressure of liquid at --------- and -- °C are ------------and -- mm. Hg respectively.

EXERCISE NO. 7.3

To determine the vapor pressure of benzene at different temperature using
Ramsay-Young apparatus

Purpose

- To learn the handing of this apparatus and determination of vapor pressure using this apparatus.
- To compare the result with the standard value at specific temperature.

Requirements

Chemicals/reagents

- Benzene
- Mercury
- Distilled water
- Other substances

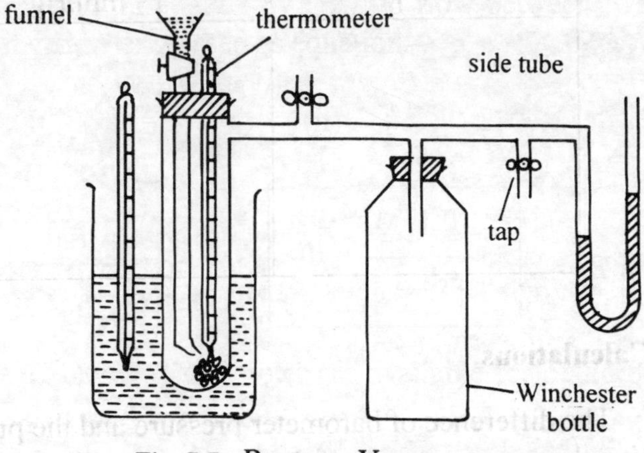

Equipments/glasswares

- Beaker
- Conical flask
- Distillation assembly
- Thermometer
- Ramsay-Young apparatus
- Winchester bottle
- Manometer
- Vacuum pump or suction pump

Fig. 7.5. Ramsay-Young apparatus.

Procedure

1. Arrange the apparatus as shown in the Fig.7.5.
2. Air tight apparatus and fill the purified water in the water bath.
3. Fill the liquid (benzene) in the dropping funnel.
4. Adjust the pressure in the apparatus 20-30 mm Hg by employing vacuum pump.
5. The height of the manometer should be adjusted to 20-30 mm.
6. Add drops of liquid by the dropping funnel on to the cotton wool surrounding the thermometer.
7. The liquid evaporates and the temperature of the liquid falls and eventually it reaches at a steady value.
8. Record the thermometer and manometer reading and determine the vapor pressure of the liquid using the equation 7.5.

9. Slowly allow air to enter into the apparatus by opening the stopcock so that the pressure inside the apparatus reaches at 50 mm Hg.

10. Repeat the step 6 to 9.

Observations

Barometer reading (atmospheric pressure) = P_1 mm. Hg

Observation table

Temperature (°C)	Manometer reading P_2 mm.Hg	Vapor pressure p $(P_1 - P_2)$ mm.Hg

Calculations

The difference of barometer pressure and the pressure difference of the manometer give the vapor pressure of the liquid at equilibrium temperature.

Vapor pressure of liquid at $T°_1$ = Barometer reading − Manometer reading

Calculate the value log p and plotted the graph between log p and 1/ T. It is represented a straight line. Determine the temperature at which the vapor pressure of the liquid is p = 760 mm, by extrapolating the graph.

Result

The vapor pressure of liquid at --------- and -- °C are ------------and -- mm. Hg respectively.

EXERCISE NO. 7.4

To determine the vapor pressure of carbon tetrachloride using as isoteniscope.

Purpose

- To learn the handling of isoteniscope and method of determination of the vapor pressure
- To familiarize the student with this apparatus and importance of the vapor pressure

Requirements

Chemicals/reagents

- Carbon tetrachloride
- Mercury
- Distilled water
- Other substances

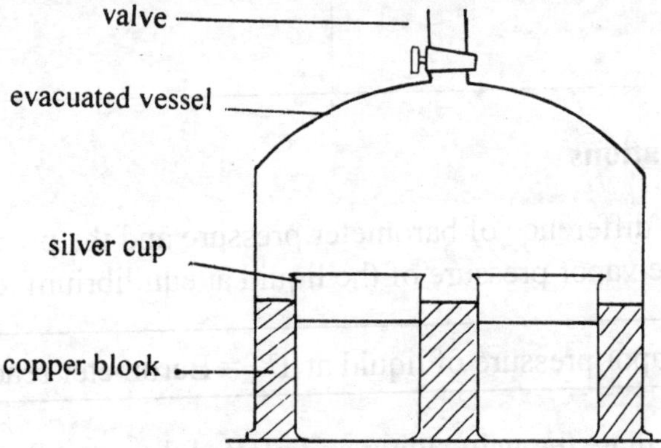

Fig. 7.6. Isopiestic apparatus

Equipments/glasswares

- Beaker
- Conical flask
- Thermometer
- Isoteniscope apparatus
- Winchester bottle
- Manometer
- Vacuum pump or suction pump

Procedure

1. Arrange the apparatus as shown in the Fig. 7.6.
2. Air tight the apparatus and fill the purified water in the water bath.
3. Fill the carbon tetrachloride in the bulb and the U-tube and test the apparatus for leaks.
4. Place the apparatus in an ice bath at about 0°C.
5. Evacuate the system so that the liquid in bulb starts to boil and air is removed from the apparatus.
6. Slowly allow the air to enter into the system so that the liquid levels in the U-tube should be the same.
7. Record the temperature and manometer reading carefully.
8. Raise the temperature of the bath and maintain it and allow air to pass by the pening D slowly until liquid levels in U-tube are same.

9. Record the temperature of bath and manometer level.

Observations

Barometer reading (atmospheric pressure) = P_1 mm. Hg

Observation table

Temperature (°C)	Manometer reading P_2 mm.Hg	Vapor pressure p $(P_1 - P_2)$ mm.Hg

Calculations

The difference of barometer pressure and the pressure difference of the manometer give the vapor pressure of the liquid at equilibrium temperature.

Vapor pressure of liquid at $T°_1$ = Barometer reading − Manometer reading

Calculate the value log p and plot the graph between log p and 1/ T. It will show a straight line. Determine the temperature at which the vapor pressure of the liquid is p = 760 mm, by extrapolating the graph.

Result

The vapor pressure of liquid at --------- and -- °C are ------------and -- mm. Hg respectively.

Viva-voce Question Bank

(a) Short answer type

1. What is vapor pressure?
2. What is osmotic pressure?
3. Give factors affecting vapor pressure.
4. How to determine the vapor pressure?
5. What is the effect of temperature on the vapor pressure?
6. Why are you determining the vapor pressure?
7. How to decrease the vapor pressure of organic solvents?
8. What is the basic principle of vapor pressure determination?
9. What is difference between vapor pressure and osmotic pressure?
10. What is manometer and barometer?

(b) State true/false

1. The vapor pressure of a liquid increases with decrease in the temperature.
2. Vapor pressure and boiling point both are same at room temperature.
3. Vapor pressure of liquid is determined by the Henry's law.
4. Clausius-Clapeyron equation is used to determine the vapor pressure.
5. Graph between vapor pressure and temperature always shows straight line.
6. Graph between Log p and 1/T is shows a straight line.
7. Every solid and liquid possesses a vapor pressure, which is a measure of the tendency of the substance to evaporate.
8. Vapor pressure of liquid is determined by static method and dynamic method.
9. Ramsay and Young's apparatus is used for the determination of vapor pressure.
10. Smith and Menzies isoteniscope is used for the determination of osmosis.

Answer (b) State true/false

    1. F   2. F   3. F   4. T   5. F   6. T   7. T   8. T   9. T   10. F

❏❏❏

Chapter 8

PARTITION COEFFICIENT

When an excess amount of solid or liquid is added to a mixture of two immiscible liquids while this substance is slightly soluble in both immiscible liquids. It will distribute itself between the two phases until saturation if mixed by shaking vigorously. If the insufficient amount of substance is added in two immiscible liquids to the saturation, it gets distributed in two layer at a definite ratio, this phenomanon is called as distribution law or partition law. The ratio constant is called as partition coefficient or distribution coefficient. It is independent of the total amount of the substance dissolved.

It was observed that if the solute has equal molecular weight in both solvents then the ratio of the concentration of the solute in the two immiscible solvent is found to be constant.

$$ K = \frac{C_1}{C_2} \qquad\qquad \text{--- (8.1)} $$

where, K is a constant known as distribution or partition coefficient. C_1 and C_2 are the concentrations of a solute in the two immiscible liquids. The concentration can be represented in g/litre or gram equivalent/liter.

Following conditions are essential for the distribution coefficients.

1. Temperature and pressure should be maintained for the solubility of a substance.Distribution of the solute in both liquids should be good and follow equation (as given above) for ideally dilute solutions.
2. Mutual solubility in two liquids must be same while adding any amount of the solute.

3. This law is only suitable for those substances which are distributed in both liquid phases and have no chemical changes like dissociation, association, degradation, hydrolysis, complex formation or any salt formation etc.

Distribution Law in Special Cases

Case I : Dissociation of solute in one of the solvent (phase)

If the solute dissociates in (1) solvent and consider the degree of dissociation as α.

Let the total concentration of the solute in solvent (1) = C_1

Therefore the concentration of the undissociated solute $= (1 - \alpha) C_1$

Now the partition coefficient on the basis of the definition

$$K = \frac{(1 - \alpha) C_1}{C_2} \qquad \text{--- (8.2)}$$

Where C_2 represents the concentration of the solute in solvent (2).

Case II : Association of solute in one of the solvent (phase)

Let the solute be associated in one of the Solvents (1) while it has normal molecular weight to the second solvent (2). Consider a reaction for the calculation of the partition coefficient.

$$nX \rightleftharpoons X_n \qquad \text{--- (8.3)}$$

Initially	1	0
After time t	$1 - \alpha$	α
Concentration	$(1 - \alpha)C_1$	αC_1

Applying law of mass action in the equation no. 8.3.

$$K_a = \frac{\alpha C_1 / n}{[(1 - \alpha)C_1]^n} \qquad \text{--- (8.4)}$$

or $\qquad (1 - \alpha)C_1 = [\alpha C_1 / n K_a]^{1/n}$

Putting this value in eq. 8.2

$$[\alpha C_1 / n K_a]^{1/n}/C_2 = K \qquad \text{--- (8.5)}$$

If solute almost dissociate completely then $\alpha \approx 1$

Now eq.8.5 $\qquad (C_1)^{1/n}/C_2 = K' \qquad \text{--- (8.6)}$
where K' is a new constant.

Case III : Solvation of solute in one of the solvent (phase)

For solving this type of problem, Let n molecules of the solvent (1) mixed with to one molecule of the solute, in ideal condition. C_1 and C_2 as the concentrations of solute in two phases.

Suppose C_3 and C_s be the concentration of the solvent molecules and the solvent molecule in the solvent (1) respectively

For one phase,

$$A + ns = A.ns \qquad\qquad \text{--- (8.7)}$$

Applying law of mass action

$$K_a = C_3 / C_1 \times C_s^n \qquad\qquad \text{--- (8.8)}$$

As N and C_s both are constant in the eq. 8.8, one can write this equation with a new constant such as.

$$C_3 / C_1 = K_a / C_s^n$$

Or $\qquad\qquad C_3 / C_1 = K' \qquad\qquad\qquad \text{--- (8.9)}$

Or $\qquad\qquad C_3 / C_1 + 1 = K' + 1$

Or $\qquad\qquad (C_1 + C_3) / C_1 = K' + 1 = K'' \qquad\qquad \text{--- (8.10)}$

According to law of distribution, $[C_1 / C_2 = K]$ eq. 8.10 written as

$$(C_1 + C_3) / C_2 = K.K''$$

or $\qquad\qquad \boxed{(C_1 + C_3) / C_2 = k} \qquad\qquad \text{--- (8.11)}$

where $(C_1 + C_3)$ is the total concentration of the solute present in the solvent phase 1, it can be determined by the analysis. K.K" is the product of two constant, i.e. equal to a new constant, k.

EXERCISE NO. 8.1

To determine the partition coefficient of iodine between carbon tetrachloride and distilled water

Purpose

- To learn method of determination of distribution coefficient and its importance in the dosage form.

Requirements

Chemicals/reagents

- Carbon tetrachloride
- Iodine
- Distilled water

Equipments/glasswares

- Separating funnel
- Conical flask
- Burette
- Pipette
- Reagent bottles

Procedure

1. Prepare a saturated solution of iodine in carbon tetrachloride (stock solution).
2. Take three reagent bottles and clean these bottles by reagent and rinse with it distilled water.
3. Prepare composition of the solution as given in the table.
4. Transfer these solution in clean and dry reagent bottles and be it as A, B, and C respectively.
5. Place the stopper on each bottle and shake it for 30 min. or shake using wrist action shaker and rotatary shaker.
6. Variability of the result depends on the shaking hence more and effective shaking is essential for reproducible results.
7. Now take this mixture in separating funnel and keep aside for about to 30 min.
8. Separate carbon tetrachloride and aqueous layer in two conical flasks.
9. Intermediate liquid can not be collected as it contain little of both liquids.
10. Put the label on both conical flasks with the samples taken originally.
11. Pipette out 10 ml of the aqueous layer and transfer in another conical flask.

12. Add 2 to 3 drops of starch solution and titrate it against 0.01 sodium thiosulphate solution.
13. Record the titration value and repeat the steps 10 and 11.
14. Similarly, titrate the aqueous layer from other containers.
15. Pipette 10 ml of carbon tetrachloride layer in a dry and clean conical flask.
16. Add starch solution 2 to 3 drops as an indicator and estimate concentration of iodine by titration with 0.01 N sodium thiosulphate solution.
17. Repeat the step 15 and 16 till you get constant burette reading.
18. Similarly, titrate other carbon tetrachloride solution as step 15 to 17.
19. Take all readings carefully.
20. Calculate concentration of iodine in both phases, i.e. aqueous and organic phase.

Table A. Preparation of solution

S.No.	Container	Composition
1.	A	25 ml stock solution + 100 ml of distilled water
2.	B	15 ml stock solution + 10 ml pure CCl_4 +100 ml of distilled water
3.	C	5 ml stock solution + 20 ml pure CCl_4 +100 ml of distilled water

Observations

Table B. Titration of aqueous layer

S.No.	Container	Volume taken (ml)	Burette reading		Volume used of 0.01N Sod. Thiosulphate (ml)
			Initial reading	Final reading	
1.	A				V_1
2.	B				V_2
3.	C				V_3

Table C. Titration of organic layer

S.No.	Container	Volume taken (ml)	Burette reading		Volume used of 0.01N Sod. Thiosulphate (ml)
			Initial reading	Final reading	
1.	A′				V_1'
2.	B′				V_2'
3.	C′				V_3'

Calculation

(a) For aqueous layer

Concentration of iodine in container A

$$N_1 V_1 = N_2 V_2$$
$$N_1 = 0.01 \times V_2 / 10$$

Concentration of iodine in water layer (C_1)

$$C_1 = (0.01 \times V_2 \times 127) / 10 \ \text{mole / liter}$$

Similarly calculate the concentration of iodine in other flask (B and C)

(b) For organic layer

Concentration of iodine in container A′

$$N_1' V_1' = N_2' V_2'$$
$$N_1' = 0.01 \times V_2' / 10$$

Concentration of iodine in water layer (C_2)

$$C_2 = (0.01 \times V_2' \times 127) / 10 \ \text{mole/liter}$$

Similarly calculate the concentration of iodine in other flask (B′ and C′)

$$\text{Partition coefficient} \quad K = C_2 / C_1$$

Result

The partition coefficient of iodine between carbon tetrachloride and distilled water = --------.

EXERCISE NO. 8.2

To determine the partition coefficient of succinic acid between ether and distilled water

Purpose

- To learn method of determination of distribution coefficient of succinic acid and its importance in the dosage form.

Requirements

Chemicals/reagents

- Ether
- Succinic acid
- 0.05 M sodium hydroxide
- Distilled water

Equipments/glasswares

- Separating funnel
- Conical flask
- Burette
- Pipette
- Reagent bottles

Procedure

1. Take three reagent bottles and clean these bottles by reagent and rinse through the distilled water.
2. Prepare composition of the solution as given in the table.
3. Transfer these solution in clean and dry reagent bottles and fix the label A, B, and C respectively.
4. Place the stopper on each bottle and shake it for 30 min.
5. Follow steps 5 to 11 as exercise no. 8.1
6. Separate two layers by separating funnel.
7. Withdraw 10 ml sample of organic layer in conical flask.
8. Add 2 to 3 drops of phenolphthalein as an indicator and titrate it using 0.05 M NaOH.
9. Repeat the above three steps and similarly titrate with etherial layer.
10. Withdraw 10 ml of aqueous layer and follow steps 9 - 10.
11. Record all estimation values carefully.

Observations

Table A. Preparation of solution

S.No.	Container	Composition
1.	A	1.0 g of succinic acid + 50 ml of ether + 50 ml of distilled water
2.	B	1.5 g of succinic acid + 50 ml of ether + 50 ml of distilled water
3.	C	2.0 g of succinic acid + 50 ml of ether + 50 ml of distilled water

Table B. Titration of aqueous layer

S.No.	Container	Volume taken (ml)	Burette reading Initial reading	Final reading	Volume used of 0.05M Sodium hydroxide (ml)
1.	A				V_1
2.	B				V_2
3.	C				V_3

Table C. Titration of organic layer

S.No.	Container	Volume taken (ml)	Burette reading Initial reading	Final reading	Volume used of 0.05M Sodium hydroxide (ml)
1.	A'				V_1'
2.	B'				V_2'
3.	C'				V_3'

Calculation

Same as exercise no. 8.1

Result

The partition coefficient of succinic acid between ether and distilled water = --------.

EXERCISE NO. 8.3

To determine the partition coefficient of succinic acid between benzene and water

Purpose

- To learn method of determination of distribution coefficient of succinic acid.

Requirements

Chemicals/reagents

- Benzene & Succinic acid
- 0.05 M sodium hydroxide

Equipments/glasswares
   Same as exercise no. 8.2

Procedure

Same as exercise no. 8.2 (take benzene in place of ether)

Observations

Table A. Titration of aqueous layer

S.No.	Container	Volume (ml)	Burette reading		Volume used of 0.05M Sodium hydroxide (ml)
			Initial	Final	
1.	A				V_1
2.	B				V_2
3.	C				V_3

Table B. Titration of of organic layer

S.No.	Container	Volume (ml)	Burette reading		Volume used of 0.05M Sodium hydroxide (ml)
			Initial	Final	
1.	A′				V_1'
2.	B′				V_2'
3.	C′				V_3'

Calculation

Same as exercise no. 8.1

Result

The partition coefficient of succinic acid between in and distilled water = -----.

EXERCISE NO. 8.4

To determine the partition coefficient of benzoic acid in benzene and distilled water

Purpose

- To learn importance and method of determination partition coefficient

Requirements

Chemicals/reagents

- Benzene
- Benzoic acid
- 0.05 M sodium hydroxide
- Distilled water

Equipments/glasswares

- Separating funnel
- Conical flask
- Burette
- Pipette
- Reagent bottles

Procedure

1. Take five reagent bottles and clean these bottles by reagent and rinse through the distilled water.
2. Prepare composition of the solution as given in the table A.
3. Transfer these solutions in clean and dry reagent bottles and place the lavel 1, 2, 3, 4 and 5 respectively.
4. Place the stopper on each bottle and shake it for 30 min.
5. Follow steps 5 to 11 as exercise no. 8.1
6. Separate two layers by separating funnel.
7. Withdraw 10 ml sample of organic layer and in conical flask.
8. Add 2 to 3 drops of phenolphthalein as indicator and titrate it using 0.05 M NaOH.
9. Repeat the procedure at least three times for accuracy and confirm reproducible results.
10. Withdraw 10 ml of aqueous layer and follow steps 9 and 10.
11. Record all estimation values carefully.

Observations

Table A. Preparation of solution

S.No.	Container	Composition
1.	1	1.0 g of benzoic acid + 50 ml of benzene + 50 ml of water
2.	2	1.5 g of benzoic acid + 50 ml of benzene + 50 ml of water
3.	3	2.0 g of benzoic acid + 50 ml of benzene + 50 ml of water
4.	4	3.0 g of benzoic acid + 50 ml of benzene + 50 ml of water
5.	5	4.0 g of benzoic acid + 50 ml of benzene + 50 ml of water

Table B. Titration of aqueous layer

S.No.	Container	Volume taken (ml)	Burette reading		Volume used of 0.05M Sodium hydroxide (ml)
			Initial reading	Final reading	
1.	A_1				V_1
2.	B_2				V_2
3.	C_3				V_3
4.	D_4				V_5
5.	E_5				V_5

Table C. Titration of organic layer

S.No.	Container	Volume taken (ml)	Burette reading		Volume used of 0.05M Sodium hydroxide (ml)
			Initial reading	Final reading	
1.	A'_1				V_1'
2.	B'_2				V_2'
3.	C'_3				V_3'
4.	D'_4				V_4'
5.	E'_5				V_5'

Calculation

Calculate the concentration of benzoic acid in benzene (organic layer) C_{org} and in distilled water (aqueous layer) C_{aqs} same as exercise no. 8.1

S.No.	Container	Concentration in organic layer (C_{org})	Concentration in aqueous layer (C_{aqs})	Partition Coefficient K (C_{org}/C_{aqs})	$\sqrt{C_{org}}/C_{aqs}$
1.	A_1/A'_1				
2.	B_2/B'_2				
3.	C_3/C'_3				
4.	D_4/D'_4				
5.	E_5/E'_5				

Result

The partition coefficient of benzoic acid in benzene and distilled water = -----.
Plot the graph between log C_{aqs} against log C_{org}, and determine the value of n and K by straight line.

Note : If the ratio of C_{org}/C_{aqs} changes with the concentration, it shows that the acid has different molecular weight in two different phases while the ratio $\sqrt{C_{org}}/C_{aqs}$ is generally constant for different concentration. It shows that benzoic acid undergoes association with benzene due to formation of dimer (combination of the two molecules of the acid).

Viva-voce Question Bank

(A) Short answer type question

1. What is distribution coefficient?
2. How to determine distribution coefficient?
3. Give factors affecting partition coefficient.
4. What is the role of partition coefficient in the dosage formulation.
5. What is the role of partition coefficient in the absorption?
6. How partition coefficient can vary?
7. What is the role of partition coefficient in the distribution?
8. What is the role of temperature in the determination of partition coefficient?
9. Give unit of partition coefficient.
10. Why you should know study partition coefficient of a drug?

(B) State true/false

1. Distribution coefficient and partition coefficient has slight difference at 55°C.
2. Distribution law is strictly applicable only in concentrated solution.
3. Benzoic acid is dimerization.
4. The substances which are not associated or not dissociated, the distribution is known true distribution coefficient.
5. The entropy of fusion and partion coefficient can be estimated from the chemical structures of the compound.

Answer (B) State true/false

1. F   2. F   3. T   4. T   5. T

◻◻◻

Chapter 9

PHASE RULE

J.Willard Gibbs studied miscibility of liquid and gaves a rule known as phase rule. It is important for the determination of least number of independent variables (temperature, pressure and concentration) affecting various phases like solid, liquid and gases. The phase rule is expressed as

$$F = C - P + 2$$

where, F is the number of degree of freedom of system, C is the number of component and P is the number of phases.

Phase is a homogeneous system which is physically district portion of a system. It is separated from other portions of a system by a boundary. If a system contain water and vapor phase. Then it is known as two phase system while mixture of ice, water and vapor is known as three phase system.

Number of component is the smallest number of constituents that participate in the formulations of phase at equilibrium e.g. at equilibrium mixture of ice, water and water vapor is in one phase because chemical formula of all three phases is H_2O.

Degree of freedom is the least number of variable which affect the phases of liquids like temperature, pressure, concentration, refractive index, density, viscosity etc. Solubility of liquids in liquids is mainly of three types

1. Completely miscible liquids
2. Partially miscible liquids
3. Immiscible liquids

When two partially miscible liquids are mixed together and mixed properly by the wrist action or vertex the tube, two different type of compositions of the liquid are obtained. Consider an example, when phenol and water are mixed mix and shakn it , two layer system is obtained upper layer is the solution of water in phenol while in lower layer is of phenol in water. At a specific temperature the combination of the both solution is fixed and both solution are in the equilibrium position. When temperature is increased, at a particular temperature or above that temperature both liquids are miscible in all proportions.

The temperature at which two partially miscible liquids are state in one phase is known as critical solution temperature.
As in this particular condition the mutual solubility increases with increasing the temperature is also known as upper consolute temperature.

In few cases like triethylamine and water, the mutual solubility increases with decreasing the temperature until a temperature is reached at which the liquids are miscible in all proportions. In such cases the curve is reverse of the phenol water system. The lowest point at which maximum solubility occurs is called as lower critical solution temperature (Fig. 9.2).

In another case like nicotine and water system, there exists both higher and lower critical solution temperature and the curve obtained is in closed form (Fig. 9.3).

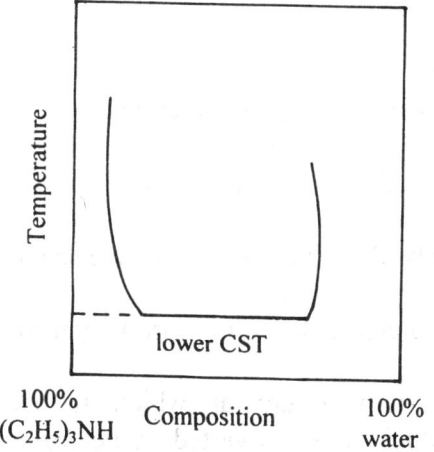

Fig. 9.2. Triethnolamine - water system.

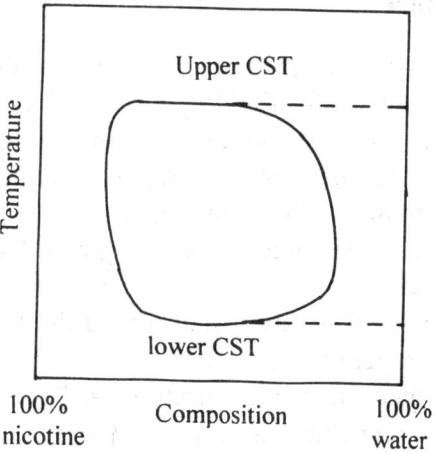

Fig. 9.3. Nicotine-water system.

EXERCISE NO. 9.1

To determine critical solution temperature of phenol and water

Purpose

- To learn the biphasic system and its importance in pharmaceutical sciences

Requirements

Chemicals/reagents

- Phenol
- Distilled water

Equipments/glasswares

- Boiling tube
- Water jacket
- Beaker
- Burette stand
- Thermometer
- Stirrer

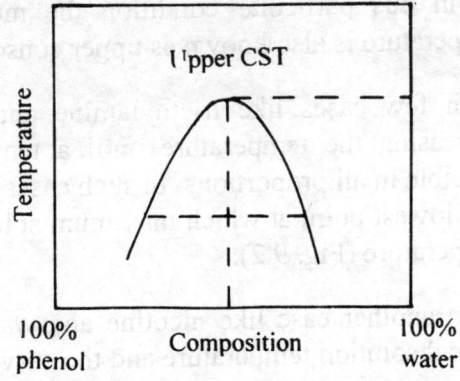

Fig. 9.1. Phenol-water system.

Procedure

(c) Arrange the apparatus as shown in the Fig. 9.4. This apparatus consist of inner tube and outer tube, fitted by the cork. Inner tube consists of thermometer and stirrer.

(d) Take 7 g of phenol in the inner tube and add exactly 7 ml of the distilled water.

(e) The mixture is mixed properly and heated gradually with continuous stirring without touching the thermometer.

(f) Note temperature at which phenol completely dissolves and is converted in one phase.

(g) Now cool it slowly and record the temperature at which the mixture is converted in heterogeneous phase.

(h) Further heat the mixture and record the temperature at which it becomes homogeneous and cooling temperature at which it is converted in heterogeneous phase.

(i) Now add 2 ml of distilled water in this test tube.

(j) Repeat steps 4 to 9.

(k) In the same tube further add 2 ml of distilled water and report the temperature at which it shows transitory opalescence.

Observations

(a) Weight of phenol   = 7.0 g.
(b) Density of distilled water at room temperature = 1 g/cm^3 (considered)
(c) Room temperature   = t °C

Observation table

S.No.	Weight of water (g.)	Percent of phenol	Temperature (°C)		
			Opalescence disappeared	Opalescence appeared	Mean value
1.	7				
2.	9				
3.	11				
4.	13				
5.	15				

Calculation

Percent of phenol = [weight of phenol/(weight of phenol +weight of water)] × 100

Plot a graph between phenol and distilled water. The curve is obtained the mutual solubility curve of phenol water system. The temperature at which it exhibits has maximum solubility, is known as critical solution temperature.

Result

The critical solution temperature of phenol-water system = ------ °C.

EXERCISE NO. 9.2

To study the effect of substances on the solubility of two immiscible liquids

Purpose

- To learn the effect of salt on the solubility of the two partially miscibility liquids

Requirements

Chemicals/reagents

- Sodium chloride solution
- Naphthalene solution
- Succinic acid
- Phenol
- Distilled water

Equipments/glasswares

- Boiling tube
- Water jacket
- Beaker
- Burette stand
- Thermometer
- Stirrer

Procedure

1. Arrange the apparatus as shown in the Fig. 9.4.
2. Take three sets of apparatus of same type.
3. Proceed as exercise no. 9.1
4. Prepare solution of 1.0% each of sodium chloride, naphthalene solution and succinic acid.
5. Add 1ml, 2 ml, ---and 5 ml of these solutions.
6. Note temperature at which phenol is completely dissolve and converted in one phase.
7. Now cool it slowly and record the temperature at which the mixture is convert in heterogeneous phase.
8. Further heat the mixture and record the temperature at which it becomes homogeneous and cool temperature at which it is converted in heterogeneous phase.
9. Add 2 ml of distilled water in this test tube.
10. Repeat steps 4 to 9.

11. In the same further add 2 ml of distilled water and report the temperature at which it shows transitory opalescence.

Observations

    (a) Weight of phenol   = 7.0 g.
    (b) Weight of distilled water   = 5.0 ml
    (c) Density of distilled water at room temperature = 1 g/cm^3 (considered)
    (d) Density of sodium chloride solution (1.0%) = -----
    (e) Density of naphthalene solution (1.0) = -------
    (f) Density of succinic acid solution (1.0) = -------
    (g) Room temperature   = t °C

Observations

Observation table

S.No.	Type of liquid		Percent of phenol	Temperature (°C)		
				Opalescence disappeared	Opalescence appeared	Mean value
1.	Water	5				
2.	Sod. Chloride	2				
3.		4				
4.		-				
5.	naphthalene	2				
6.		4				
7.		-				
8.	succinic acid	2				
9		4				
10.		-				

Calculation

Percent of phenol = [weight of phenol/(weight of phenol +weight of liquids)] × 100

Result

    The critical solution temperature of phenol-water system = ---,---and,--- °C.

EXERCISE NO. 9.3

To determine the composition and the amount of layer obtained by mixing phenol and distilled water in equal proportion

Purpose

- To learn method of determination of composition of any liquid at a specific temperature.

Requirements

Chemicals/reagents

- Phenol
- Distilled water

Equipments/glasswares

Same experiment no. 9.1

Procedure

1. Take 45 g of phenol and 55 g of distilled water in a boiling tube
2. Proceed as in exercise no. 9.1.
3. On the basis of the observation, plot a tie, line.
4. The composition of the liquid is measured by the Lever rule.

Observations

Same as in exercise no.9.1.

Calculation

Using Lever rule for determination of the composition

$$W_1 / W_2 = XL_1 / XL_2$$
$$\text{As} \quad W_1 + W_2 = 100$$
$$\text{Hence,} \quad W_1 / (100 - W_1) = XL_1 / XL_2$$

Where, L_1 & L_1 are left hand right hand layers, X intersection point and W_1 & W_2 are the weight of two layers.

Result

On the basis of graph, composition of the two layers is determined at t °C

EXERCISE NO. 9.4

To study a solubility curve of a ternary system

Purpose

- To learn concept of the ternary system and its importance.

Requirements

Chemicals/reagents

- Acetic acid & chloroform

Equipments/glasswares

Same as in exercise 9.1

Procedure

1. Prepare solution of acetic acid and chloroform.
2. Take four bottles and prepare the solution on the basis of the percentage composition by weight of the chloroform (10, 20, 40, and 80%).
3. Density of acetic acid is 1.05 while density of chloroform is 1.50 g/ml.
4. Composition of the solution is given in table A.
5. Add distilled water in small quantity in each container.
6. Shake the container, an appearance of the turbidity indicates that the system is heterogeneous.

Observations

Table A. Composition of solution

Sen.	Container	Acetic acid (ml)	Chloroform (ml)
1.	A	21.4	1.7
2.	B	19.1	3.3
3.	C	14.3	6.7
4.	D	4.8	13.3

Table B. Observations

S.No	Volume of acetic acid (ml)	Volume of chloroform (ml)	Volume of water (ml)	Percent by weight of acetic acid	Percent by weight of chloroform	Percent by weight of water
1.	21.4	1.7				
2.	19.1	3.3				
3.	14.3	6.7				
4.	4.8	13.3				
5.						

Calculation

Variation in the miscibility limits with the composition of the three component systems is shown in the form of triangular diagram.

Result

Solubility curve of the ternary system is shown in the graphical form.

Viva- voce Question Bank

1. What is phase rule?
2. What is Lever rule?
3. What is the importance of the phase rule?
4. Define binary system.
5. Explain ternary phase with suitable examples.
6. Give applications of the binary phase in manufacturing.
7. How to measure the binary system?
8. What is critical solution temperature?
9. How to determine CST?
10. What is tie line?
11. Give factors effecting the tie line.

Chapter 10

COLLOIDS

On the basis of diffusion of substances through the semi-permeable membrane, Thomas Grahms classified the substances into two categories.

1. Crystalloids (having higher rate of diffusion)
2. Colloids (having slow rate of diffusion)

The term colloid has been derived from Greek word 'Kolla' means glue and 'iods' means like, hence colloids are those substance which have glue like nature. Colloidal systems are defined as polyphasic systems in which disperse phase particles measures between 10-1000 A°.

Characteristics of colloidal state

1. Colloidal state contains at least two phases, the one phase dispersed in other is called as internal phase or dispersed phase and the media in which it is dispersed is called as a dispersion medium.
2. Particle size of colloidal state is an intemediate between true solution and suspension state.
3. Colloidal particles can not be detected under ordinary microscope and required ultramicroscope.
4. Colloidal state particles can diffuse through parchment membrane slowly.
5. The surface area of colloidal state particle is very large.
6. Colloidal particle always carry charge (+)ve or (-)ve on dispersed phase particles.
7. Colloidal particles do not settle under the force of gravity.

Classification of Colloids

Many methods are used for the classification of colloidal dispersion. It can be classified on the basis of dispersion medium, charge it posses and affinity of dispersion phase for dispersion medium.

1. On the basis of Dispersion Medium

    (a) Hydrosols (if dispersion medium is water)
    (b) Alcosols (if dispersion medium is alcohol)
    (c) Benzosols (if dispersion medium is benzene)
    (d) Aerosols (if dispersion medium is air)

2. On the basis of charge

    (a) Positive sols
    (b) Negative sols

3. On the basis of affinity of dispersion phase for dispersion medium

    (a) Lyophilic colloids
    (b) Lyophobic colloids

Property	Lyophilic sols	Lyophobic sols
Nature	Disperse phase has more affinity for aqueous phase	has less affinity
Preparation	Easily prepared	Need special methods
Concentration of sol	More concentration of disperse phase in the sol	Less concentration of disperse phase in the sol
Stability	More stable	Less stable
Size of sol particle	Small	Large
Viscosity	More viscous than dispersion medium	Same as dispersion medium
Surface tension	Less than dispersion medium	Same as dispesion medium
Reversibility	It is reversible with temperature	Not reversible with temp.
Charge	Charge on sol particles depends upon pH of medium	Charge on sol particles not depends upon pH of medium
Tyndall effect	Exhibits less scattering effect	Exhibits more scattering effect
Solvation	Posses high degree of solvation	Posses low degree of solvation

METHOD OF PREPARATION

Lyophilic sols are easily formed as contact disperse phase comes in contact with dispersion medium. However special methods are required to prepare lyophobic sols such as

1. Dispersion method

- Grinding method
- Peptization method
- Bredig arc method

2. Condensation method

A. Physical methods
- Exchange of solvent method
- Excessive cooling method
- Condensing vapor method

B. Chemical methods
- Double decomposition method
- Hydrolysis method
- Reduction method

PROPERTIES OF COLLOIDS

1. Physical properties

- Diffuse slowly through the parchament membrane.
- Easily passed through the ordinary filter papers.
- It is hetrogeneous in nature.
- Particles of sols do not settle down by the gravity.
- Viscosity and surface tension of sols are same as dispersion medium.
- Surface area of particles are very large as compared to the other heterogeneous system
- High adsorption power due to larger surface area.
- Shapes and size of sol particles are different due to different colors.

2. Colligative properties

Colloidal solutions exhibit colligative properties but slightly lesser than the true solution because in colloidal state, there exist aggregates of thousands of molecules of high molecular weight and thus number of particles being low than true solutions

- Osmotic pressure
- Elevation of boiling point
- Depression in freezing point
- Lowering in vapor pressure

3. Optical properties

- When a beam of light is passed through the colloidal solution, a visible cone is observed due to the scattering of light by the colloidal particles, this phenomenon is known as *Faraday- Tyndall effect.*
- The size, shape and structure of colloidal particles is observed by the *electron microscope* because it has high resolving power.
- All colloidal solutions exhibits *scattering of light* or opalescence.

4. Kinetic properties

- Colloidal particles posses irregular or chaotic motion like pollen grains when suspended in water, such motion is known as Brownian motion because it is observed by Robert Brown.
- Colloidal particles are diffused continuously from a region of higher concentration to one of the lower concentration until the system achieve concentration uniformly. It can be determined by the Fick's first law

$$\frac{dq}{dt} = -DS\frac{dc}{dx}$$

where dq/dt rate of diffusion, D is the diffusion coefficient, dc/dx is the concentration gradient, and S is the surface area of diffusion.

- Van't Hoff equation is used to calculate the molecular weight of a colloid solution in dilute state.

$$\frac{\pi}{c_g} = \frac{RT}{M}$$

- If the colloidal particles are subjected only to the force of gravity, then the lower size of particles obeying Stoke's law.

$$v = \frac{2r^2(\rho - \rho_0)g}{9\eta_0}$$

where, ρ - density of disperse particles, ρ_0 - density of dispersion medium,
v - velocity of sedimentation and η_0 - viscosity of the dispersion medium.

5. Electrical properties

- Colloidal particles always posses positive or negative charge, absence of charge on the dispersed phase particles result in unstability colloidal solutions. The origin of charge on the sol particles have been explained on the basis of the following concepts.
  (i) Charge due to fraction
  (ii) Capture of electron by the sol particles
  (iii) Nature of dispersed phase
  (iv) Groups present on the dispersed phase
  (v) Charge to ion adsorption
- Helmholtz gave electrical double layer concept for the distribution of charge on the colloidal particles and gave the utility of electrostatic charge and zeta potential on the stability of the sols.

Some Important Terminology

Cataphoresis : The migration of colloidal particles under the influence of electrical field is known as cataphoresis or electrophoresis.

Electro Osmosis : The movement of the dispersion medium under the influence of electrical field is known as electro osmosis while dispersed phase particles are inhibited to move.

Coagulation : Spontaneous breaking up of a colloidal solution and separation of dispersed phase from the dispersion medium is called as aging and phenomenon is known as coagulation.

Gold number : Gold number of a lyophilic subtance is defined as the minimum amount of lyophilic subtance in milligrams which prevents the coagulation of 10 ml gold sol against the addition of 10% of sodium chloride solution. Higher is the gold number, lesser is the protective power of lyophilic colloid. Gold number of some protective colloids are acacia (0.1-0.2), albumin (0.1), gelatin (0.005- 0.01), sodium oleate (1.0-5.0), and tragacanth (2.0).

Micelle : The aggregation of ions of colloids or molecules to form sol particles is known as the micelle. The minimum concentration of surfactant at which micelle formation starts is known as critical miscelle concentration (CMC). If the CMC formation require lesser amount of surfactant, it is concluded that it has more surface activity and high detergency.

Detergents : Substances which have surface activity as well as cleaning action is known as detergents.

Surfactants : The substances which have capacity to reduce the surface tension of liquids or tendency to increase surface area and posses surface activity is called as surfactants.

Gels : Dispersion of liquid in solid are known as gels. If it contains higher dispersion medium, it is known as jellies. Gels are unstable and stabilized by the gelling agent. Separation of internal liquid from the gels without disturbing the basic structure of gels, is known as syneresis or weeping of gels.

Nernst potential : It is defined as the potential difference between the actual surface and the electroneutral region of the colloidal solution.

Zeta potential : Zeta potential is the difference in electrical potential between a tightly bound layer of ions on particle surfaces and the bulk liquid in which the particles are suspended.

$$\zeta = \frac{v}{E} \times \frac{4\pi\eta}{\varepsilon} \times 9 \times 10^4$$

Where ζ is the zeta potential in volts, v migration velocity of sol particles in cm/sec., η the viscosity of the medium in poises (dyne sec/cm^2), ε dielectric constant of the medium and the potential gradient E in the volts/cm. The ratio of v/E is known as the *mobility*. The stability of dispersed system depends on the zeta potential. If the zeta potential is reduced below a certain limit, the attractive force between particles exceeds than the repulsive forces and particles come together. Attraction of particles and formation of coagulate is known as flocculation.

Krafft point : The temperature at which the solubility of the surfactant equals the critical micelle concentration is known as krafft point.

Cloud point : The temperature at which the separation of surfactants occurs as a precipitates due to self association and loss of water of hydration of individual molecules in the solution.

EXERCISE NO. 10.1

To prepare and study colloidal solution of arsenic sulphide

Purpose

- To familiarize colloid and its method of preparation.
- To learn stability and purification of colloidal solution.
- To learn importance and pharmaceutical application of colloid.

Requirements

Chemicals/reagents
- Arsenic oxide
- Distilled water
- Ferric sulphide
- Dilute sulphuric acid
- Hydrogen sulphide gas
- Soda lime

Equipments/glasswares

- Instrument of hydrogen sulphide (Kipp's apparatus)
- Round bottom flask
- Beaker
- Plastic tube
- Parchment paper

Procedure

1. Weigh100 g of pure arsenic oxide and heat it in 200 ml of distilled water till it dissolved.
2. Cool this solution at room temperature.
3. If arsenic oxide is not dissolved completely then filter it and get a clear solution at room temperature.
4. Pass the hydrogen sulphide* (H_2S) into this solution till the opalescent liquid becomes yellow turbid.
5. Excess of hydrogen sulphide gas is removed by passing a stream of carbon dioxide (CO_2) or hydrogen gas through this solution.

---

* Hydrogen sulphide should be washed by bubbling through water two to three time.

6. Filter the sol through filter paper to remove the coarse precipitate of arsenic sulphide and collect the filterate sol in the separate beaker.
7. This sol contains impurities of electrolytes and other soluble substances. It can be removed by dialysis*.
8. Fill the sol in parchment bag and hang in the beaker which contain distilled water. It can be changed after some time or regularly.
9. Dialysis process can be enhanced by applying an electric field using electrode[#].
10. After dialysis it will give a pure arsenic sulphide sol.
11. Performe necessary test for this sol like optical and kinetic properties of sols.

Observations

- Following tests are performed after preparation of sol
- Uniformity of sol particles by electron microscopy
- Sedimentation of particles
- Charge of sol
- Density of sol
- Optical characteristics
- Brownian motion
- Stability

Result
Prepared sol of arsenic sulphide is uniform and shows all characteristics of colloids

---

* The colloidal solution prepared by any method, contains impurities of electrolyte and some impurities of other soluble substances which may get precipitated on standing of the colloidal solution. These impurities are removed by subjecting the sol through a process iknown as dialysis.

[#] Dialysis process may be enhanced by employing an electric field, such process is known as ectrodialysis.

EXERCISE NO. 10.2

To prepare and study colloidal solution of ferric hydroxide

Purpose

- To prepare and learn utility of ferric hydroxide sol

Requirements

Chemicals/reagents

- Ferric chloride
- Ammonium carbonate
- Distilled water

<u>*Equipments/glasswares*</u>

Same as given in exercise no. 10.1

Procedure

1. Prepare saturated solution of ferric chloride* in distilled water in beaker.
2. Boil 250 ml of distilled water in a separate beaker.
3. Add dropwise saturated solution of ferric chloride in the boiled water with continuous stirring.
4. Ferric chloride solution is hydrolysed and form a deep red sol of ferric hydroxide.
5. When preparing the solution add about 10 ml of 30% solution of ferric chloride in the boiling water before adding solution.
6. Dialysis the prepared sol for purification
7. Remove the chloride ions from the sol.

Observations

All parameters will be performed as given in the exercise no. 10.1.

Result

Prepared sol of arsenic sulphide is uniform and form the chloride ions. It shows all characteristics of colloids.

---

* It is not necessary to prepare saturated solution of ferric chloride. Any other concentration of the this solution can be prepared as per the instruction of teacher or study for the same

EXERCISE NO. 10.3

To prepare and study colloidal solution of silver

Purpose

- To learn method of preparation of silver sol and its advantages in the electroplating.

Requirements

Chemicals/Reagents

- Silver nitrate
- Distilled water
- Sodium carbonate

Equipments/Glasswares

Same as given in exercise no. 10.1

Procedure

1. Prepare 50 ml of 0.1M silver nitrate solution in the distilled water in 100 ml of conical flask.
2. Prepare 25ml of 1% solution of tannic acid in the distilled water in separate 100 ml of conical flask.
3. Add 20 ml nitrate solution and 10 ml of tannic acid solution in 500 ml of distilled water.
4. Heat this mixture at 75-80°C for 10 min.
5. Add 10 ml of 1% solution of sodium carbonate slowly with continuous stirring.
6. Silver carbonate is formed, it is reduced immediately by tannic acid to the metallic silver.
7. Dispersed state of silver is in tea colored.
8. Immpurities of electrolytes and soluble substances are removed by the dialysis.

Observations

(a) Colloidal solution of the silver is stable and uniformly distributed. It exhibits clear tea colored of silver sol.
(b) Other observation is the same as given in the exercise no. 10.1.

Result

Prepared sol of silver is uniform and stable. It shows all characteristics of colloids.

EXERCISE NO. 10.4

To prepare and study colloidal solution of gelatin

Purpose

- To familiarize with the colloidal state of substances and their application in this over the other state of the same substances.

Requirements

Chemicals/reagents

- Gelatin
- Distilled water

Equipments/glasswares

Same as given in the exercise no. 10.1

Procedure

1. Weigh 2.0 g of gelatin powder carefully using analytical balance or electronic single pan balance.
2. Take 500 ml of distilled water in beaker.
3. Heat the water at 80-90°C.
4. Add weighed amount of gelatin in the heated water with continuous stirring till it dissolved.
5. Cool the solution at room temperature without applying any mean of cooling*.

Observations

(a) Cool solution of gelatin at room temperature shows a clear sol of gelatin. Other parameter should be same as given in the exercise no.10.1

Result

Same as exercise no. 10.3.

---

* At higher temperature and sudden cooling and heating the solution undergoes coagulation of the gelatin. Hence it is necessary to maintain the temperature properly and take all necessary precaution for the preparation of the gelatin sol important in pharmaceutical products.

EXERCISE NO. 10.5

To study the effect of sodium chloride (monovalent), barium chloride (divalent) and aluminium chloride (trivalent) on arsenic sulphide sol.

Purpose

- To learn the factors effecting stability of the sol.
- To learn effects of salt on the sability of sol.

Requirements

Chemicals/reagents

- Prapred arsenic sulphide sol
- Sodium chloride solution
- Barium chloride solution
- Arsenic sulphide solution
- Distilled water
- Other reagents

Equipments/glasswares

- Test tubes
- Beakers
- Conical flasks
- Pipette graduated
- Bunsen burner
- Other necessary glasswares

Procedure

1. Take 20 test tubes with screw cap. Clean and dry it as per usual.
2. Fix proper label on the test tube, having mark as 1,2,3,4-----------& 30 etc. in the serial.
3. Transfer solution of sodium chloride and distilled water in two different burettge.
4. Add 1 ml, 2ml, 3ml ---------of sodium chloride solution in increasing order upto 10 ml in the test tubes. Then add 9.0 ml, 8.0 ml --------------0.0 ml of distilled water in test tube so that total volume becomes 10 ml.
5. Add 10 ml prepared sol of arsenic sulphide in each set of test tube.
6. Replaced cap of the tube and vortex or shake all test tube for a few minutes on the vortex.
7. Now allow to stand the test tube in the test tube stand for 2 h.

8. Report number of the test tube which shows turbidity and report the composition oof the same.
9. If the turbidity is found in the test tube 4 and 5, it means that the precipitation formed in the test tube between the range of 4 and 5 ml of 0.2M NaCl is precipitate of the colloids.
10. For the exact concentration determination, prepare another set of the test tube in the same way as in step 4 to 9.
11. Apply method for the solution of barium chloride and aluminium chloride using the steps 1 to 11 carefully.

Observations

(a) 0.2M solution of NaCl
(b) Arsenic sulphide solution

Table A

Test tube number	Distilled water (ml)	Quantity of 0.2M NaCl solution (ml)	Observation
1	9.0	1.0	
2	8.0	2.0	
3	7.0	3.0	
4	6.0	4.0	
5	5.0	5.0	
-	-	-	
-	-	-	
10	0.0	10.0	

Table B

Test tube number	Distilled water (ml)	Quantity of 0.2M NaCl solution (ml)	Observation
11	6.0	4.0	
12	5.9	4.1	
13	5.8	4.2	
14	5.7	4.3	
15	5.6	4.4	
-	-	-	
-	-	-	
20	5.1	4.9	
21	5.0	5.0	

Calculation

Concentration of sodium chloride in the each test tube as mentioned, 1 to 10 number can be determined by applying the following formula.

1.0 ml of 0.2 ml stock solution of NaCl have = 0.2 millimole of the salt

If this solution is diluted to 20.0 ml

Hence,

100 ml of this solution would contain = 0.2/20 × 1000 = 10.0 millimoles.

In the same method the concentration of the sodium chloride in the other 2 to 10 will be equivalent amount of sodium chloride is 20, 30, 40, -----------100.0 millimoles per liter.

In this method calculate the concentration of the other ion concentration in the different solution barium chloride and aluminium chloride.

Result

The precipitation values of various salt for arsenic sulphide sol of sodium chloride, barium chloride, and aluminium chloride are ---, --- and -----, respectively.

EXERCISE NO. 10.6

To determine the effect of potassium chloride and potassium sulphate on ferric hydroxide sols

Purpose

- To learn the factors effecting stability of the sol.
- To learn effects of salt on the sability of sol.

Requirements

Chemicals/reagents

- Prepared ferric hydroxide sol
- Potassium chloride solution
- Potassium sulphate solution
- Distilled water

Equipments/glasswares

Same as given in exercise no. 10.5.

Procedure

1. Prepare sol of ferric hydroxide.
2. Follows all steps as given in the exercise no. 10.5.

Observations

Obsretation table A

Test tube number	Distilled water (ml)	Quantity of 0.2M KCl Solution (ml)	Observation
1	9.0	1.0	
2	8.0	2.0	
3	7.0	3.0	
-	-	-	
-	-	-	
10	0.0	10.0	

Put result in the same way as exercise no.10.5

EXERCISE NO. 10.7

To study the protective action of hydrophilic colloid on the precipitaion of a hydrophobic colloid.

Purpose

- To learn the protective action of the subtances
- To familiarize with the gold number and its application in colloidal solution

Requirements

Chemicals/reagents

- Gelatin
- Albumin
- Starch
- Distilled water
- Arsenic sulphide sol
- Sodium chloride solution

Equipments/glasswares

- Beaker
- Burette
- Volumetric flask
- Funnel
- Other necessary glasswares

Procedure

1. Arrange a set of test tube having volume about 25 ml.
2. Fix proper label 1 to 10 and arrange these tube serially in a suitable rack.
3. Add 10 ml prepared sol of arsenic sulphide in each tube by burette.
4. Add (0.1%) starch solution 0, 1, 2 -----8, and 9 ml in the tube 1,2,--------9 and 10 respectively.
5. Add distilled water 10, 9, 8,-------3, 2, and 1 ml in the tube number 1, 2, 3,------9 and 10 respectively.
6. Replace cap on the tube and tight it.
7. Mix this contents by wrist action shaker or vetex or by hand so that it can be mix throughly.
8. Allow test tube to stand for 24 h. without disturbing the set of the tube.
9. After 24 h. observe the test tube in which *the* precipitation is not formed.

10. In the same way repeat step 1 to 9 using other protective agents like gelatin and alumin in the various concentration.

Observations

Observation Table*

Test tube number	Amount of sol (As_2S_3) ml	Amount of sodium chloride (ml)	Amount of distilled water (ml)	Observation
1	10	0	10	Test tube in
2	10	1	9	which no
3	10	2	8	precipitation
4	10	3	7	after 24 h.
5	10	4	6	
6	10	5	5	
7	10	6	4	
8	10	7	3	
9	10	8	2	
10	10	9	1	

Calculation

Test tube number 1 to 10 contain starch 0, 1, 2, ------------7, 8, and 9 molligrams respectively.

Determine the concentration of starch obtained from the observe the test tube which shows protective action on the sols.

Result

On the basis of observation it was found that -----milligram of starch --------milligram of gelatin and --------- milligram of albumin protect the colloid of precipitation

---

* For other substances make separate table of protective colloids like albumin and gelatin. In whole of the study use these substances in solution.

EXERCISE NO. 10.8

To determine the optimum ratio for precipitation.

Purpose

- To study the mutual coagulation of sols.
- To learn the factors affecting the precipitation.

Requirements

Chemicals/reagents

- Arsenic sulphide sol
- Ferric hydroxide sol
- Distilled water

Equipments/glasswares

- Test tube
- Test stand
- Burette
- Other necessary glasswares

Procedure

1. Prepare sol of arsenic sulphide as exercise no. 10.1.
2. Prepare sol of ferric sulphide as exercise no. 10.2.
3. Prepare a set of arrangement which contain 1 to 9 test tube.
4. Transfer 1, 2, ---- 8 and 9 ml As_2S_3 sol in each tube and then add 9, 8,-------2, and 1 ml of ferric hydroxide sol in the test tube serially.
5. Mix all test tube using vertex or wrist action shaker for a few minutes.
6. Allow to stand the test tube for about 2 h without disturbing.
7. After 2 h observe the test tube for precipitation and thus determine the optimum ratio for precipitation of these sols.
8. If consider that 9 ml of arsenic sulphide and 1 ml of ferric hydroxide sols shows the precipitation.
9. Repeat the step 3 to 7 with the quantities as given in the observation table B
10. After 2 h observe the test tubes and finally determine the concentration at which it shows precipitation using these two sols.
11. Calculate the concentration of these two sols in milligrams.
12. Report the result in the scientific manner.

Observations

Table A

Test tube number	Amount of arsenic sulphide sol (ml)	Amount of ferric hydroxide sol (ml)	Observations
1	1	9	Report the precipitation in the test tube and determine the ratio at which two sols give the precipitation
2	2	8	
3	3	7	
4	4	6	
5	5	5	
6	6	4	
7	7	3	
8	8	2	
9	9	1	

Table B

Test tube number	Amount of arsenic sulphide sol (ml)	Amount of ferric hydroxide sol (ml)	Observations
1	8.5	1.5	Report the precipitation in the test tube and determine the optimum ratio at which two sols give the precipitation
2	8.6	1.4	
3	8.7	1.3	
4	8.8	1.2	
5	8.9	1.1	
6	9.0	1.0	
7	9.1	0.9	
8	9.2	0.8	
9	9.3	0.7	
10	9.4	0.6	
11	9.5	0.5	

Calculation

Calculate the optimum ratio of two sols and their concentration at which it shows the precipitation.

Result

Two sols arsenic suphite and sodium hydroxide show the precipitation when mixed in the ----- milligrams and -------- milligrams respectively.

EXERCISE NO. 10.9

To determine the charge on the particles in a given colloidal solution
and determine zeta potential.

Purpose

- To learn mechanism of charge distribution on the sol particles.
- To study the characteristics of charge on the sol.

Requirements

Chemicals/reagents

- Arsenic sulphide sol or ferric hydroxide sol
- Potassium chloride solution
- Distilled water

Equipments/glasswares

- Electrophoresis apparatus
- Cathetometer
- Conductance bridge
- DC supply (rectifier)

Procedure

1. Arrange the assembly after cleaning it properly and check leakage any liquid if any exists in the system.
2. Check both side arms taps & knobs for any types of leakage and grease if required.
3. Fill the sol in the U-tube and open the taps of arms so that it can be partially filled in the both arms.
4. Turn off the taps and adjust the volume of the sol in both arms.
5. Fill both arms with dispersion medium (distilled water) and insert two platinum foil electrode in the dispersion medium.
6. Slowly open the tap of side arm and take care that no mixing of the sol and dispersion medium and they shows a sharp boundary between them.
7. Set a telescope of the cathetometer on one of the boundaries and adjust the height of the telescope.
8. Record the initial reading of the boundary between these two liquids.
9. Apply DC current using the electrode at potential differences of 100-150 volts.
10. Allow the current flow for about 10-15 min.
11. boundries. Record the time of supply and potential supplies accurely.
12. Record the polarity and direction of migration of the

13. At a fix time interval determine the position of the boundary using the same apparatus arrangement.
14. Calculate the distance travelled by this liquid or movement of the boundary.
15. Clean the apparatus and fill with 0.1M potassium chloride solution in the same assembly.
16. Insert the electode in both arms with the foil at the same position as arrange for sol.
17. Measure the resistance of the solution between the electrode.
18. Change the position of the electrode and determine the resistance of the new solution column.
19. Viscosity of the sol is determined by the Ostwald's viscometer.
20. Calculate the mobility using the observation datas.

Observations

Applied Potential $= V$ volts

S.No.	Initial position of the boundary	Final position of the boundary	Distance traveled by the layer x (cm)	Time of passage of current t (sec)	$v = x / t$
1.					
2.					
3.					
4.					
5.					

   (a) Resistance of potassium chloride between two the electrode $= R_1$ ohms
   (b) Distance through which the electrode move $= 1$ cm
   (c) Resistance of the fresh solution $= R_2$ ohms

Calculation

$$\text{The distance between the electrode of the foils} = \frac{1 \times R_1}{R_2 - R_2} = L \text{ cm}$$

$$\text{Potential gradient} = \frac{V}{L} = E \text{ volts/cm}$$

Zeta potential is determine by the following equation

$$\zeta = \frac{4\pi\eta v}{DE}$$

Where, η viscosity of the sol determine by the Ostvald's viscometer some time this is equal to the viscosity of the dispersion medium

(a) v is the linear velocity of the particles, determine by the observation data.
(b) D is the dielectric constant of the dispersion medium
(c) E is potential gradient

By applying this equation zeta potential is determined.

Result

    Zeta potential of the given sol was ----- volts

Viva-voce Question Bank

(A) Short answer type questions
1. What is colloid?
2. What is miscelle?
3. How to prepare colloids?
4. Give advantages of colloids.
5. What is the role of colloids in pharmaceutical dosage forms?
6. What is difference between lyophilic and lyophobic colloids?
7. Why sky appears blue?
8. How rubber is obtained by latex?
9. What is gel?
10. What is sol?
11. What is difference between emulsion and colloids?
12. What is difference between solution and colloids?
13. What is electrostatic precipitation of carbon?
14. Why medicine are more effective in the form of colloids?
15. What is difference between gels and jellies?
16. What is saponification?
17. Give examples of natural colloids.
18. What is coagulation?

(B) Define following terms with examples and their importance in the pharmacy.

i. Colloids   ii. Sols   iii. lyophilic colloids   iv. lyophobic colloids   v. association colloids

vi. micelle   vii. Tyndall effect   viii. Brownian motion   ix. Diffusion   x. Osmosis
xi. Zeta potential   xii. Nernst potential   xii. Donnan membrane   xiii. Krafft point
xiv. Cloud point   xv.Solubilization   xvi. Gold number   xvii.Schulze-Hardy rule
xviii. Protective colloids   xix. Optical properties of colloids   xx. Kinetic properties of colloids.

(C) State true/false
1. The size of colloid particles is in the range of 10^{-7} to 10^{-5} micron.
2. Colloidal particles are filtered through filter paper.
3. Milk is an emulsion.
4. Peptization is a characteristic property of sols.
5. Metal sols has (–)ve charge
6. The colour of colloidal solution is not independent of the size and shape of sols particles.
7. Colloidal silica is a protective colloid.
8. Gold number is the index for purity of gold.
9. Gelatin is generally used in making ice cream to stabilise the colloid and prevent the crystallization.
10. The crystallization power of an electrolyte is determined in the form of coagulation value.
11. Emulsion is a colloidal system of solid dispersed in liquid.
12. The capacity of an ion to coagulate a colloidal solution depends on shape of particles.
13. Ferric chloride stops bleeding due to coagulation.
14. Higher the gold number lesser is the protective power of colloids.
15. Tyndall effect is observed mainly in the sols.

Answer (A) State true/false
1. T   2. T   3. T   4. F   5. T   6. F   7. T   8. F
9. T   10. T   11. F   12. F   13. T   14. T   15. T

❑❑❑

REFRACTIVITY

The measurement of refractive index of substances is very important in physical chemistry. It gives some invaluable information about the characteristics of the compound, purity of compound, and composition of the compound.

When a monochromatic light passes from one isotopic medium to another medium, its path changes at the interfaces of the two medium. If a ray of light passes through a rarer medium to a denser medium, it deviates towards the normal at the interface and if the rays passes through a denser medium to rarer medium, it deviates away from the normal at the interface (Fig. 12.1). This phenomenon is known as refraction.

Snell's Law of Refraction

According to this law 'the ratio of sines of angle of incidence and of angle of refraction is a constant quantity is known as refraction index which is also equal to the ratio of velocity of light in the two media one is rarer and other is denser.

$$n = \frac{Sin\ i}{Sin\ r} = \frac{\text{velocity of light in one medium}}{\text{velocity of light in second medium}} \qquad \text{--- (11.1)}$$

Where, i and r are the of incidence angles and refraction angles respectively.

If the angle of incidence is increased, the angle of refraction would also increase and achieve the maximum angle (i = 90°).

$$n = \frac{Sin\ 90}{Sin\ r'} = \frac{1}{Sin\ r'}$$

The angle r' is known as the critical angle.

Measurement of Refractive Index

Main principle of refractometers are based on the critical angle. Three main instruments are generally used in the laboratory for the determination of the refractive index such as

(a)   Abbe refractometer
(b)   Pulfrich refractometer
(c)   Immersion refractometer

Abbe refractometer is commonly used in the laboratory because it have number of advantages over the other instruments available in the market, viz.

1. Small quantity of the sample is required for the analysis.
2. Convenient, simple and reliable method.
3. Covers a wide range for determination of refractive index.
4. Monocromatic light is not required for the analysis.
5. Easy method for determination of the refractive method.
6. Economic method.
7. Easy to maintain the instrument.

Abbe refractometer has mainly following parts

1. Prism box
2. Index arm
3. Telescope
4. Dispersion compensator
5. Metallic mirror

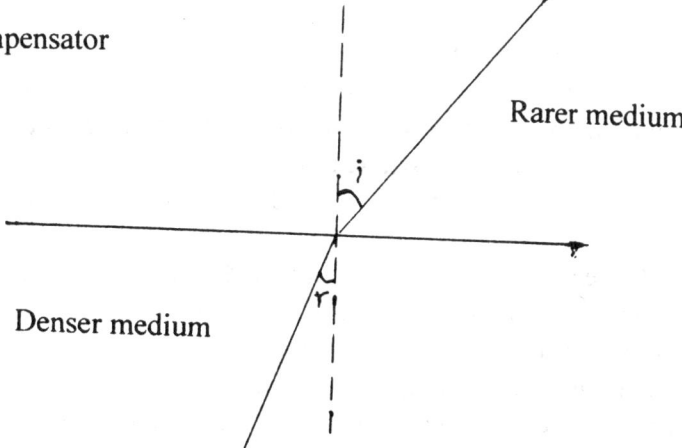

Fig. 11.1. Refrection

EXERCISE NO. 11.1

To determine refractive index of a given liquid using Abbe refractometer

Purpose

- To learn principle and handling of refractometer
- To study the refractive index and its importance in the field of pharmacy

Requirements

Chemicals/Reagents

- Sample of liquid
- Rectified spirit
- Distilled water

Equipments/Glasswares

- Abbe refractometer
- Soft brush or cotton
- Plastic pipe attachment

Procedure

1. Place the apparatus infront of proper light source.
2. Clean the apparatus using soft cloth and wipe the prism by soft brush, if necessary, moistened with alcohol and then acetone.
3. Place a drop of distilled water and adjust the instrument.
4. Focus the telescope eye piece on the cross section of the instrument and rotate the index arm until a colored band or fringe is seemed through the telescope.
5. Adjust the eye piece on the movable arm to give sharp focus on the scale and record the refractive index to the third place of decimal and for fourth place use a reading lens.
6. Take at least three reading of each sample and its mean used for calculation.
7. Open the prism by turning the lock nut and clean the faces of the prism.
8. Put a few drop test solution on prism and closed it properly.
9. Take three reading of each sample of liquid.
10. Density of liquid is determined by pycnometer or density bottle.

Observations

1.Experimental temperature = t °C
2.Refractive index of water at t °C = ------
3.Density of test liquid = ------

Observation table

S.No.	Distilled water				Liquid			
	Refractive index			Mean	Refractive index			Mean
	(a)	(b)	(c)		(a)	(b)	(c)	
1. 2. 3.								

Result

The refractive of the given liquid at temperature (room temperature) = ----------

view

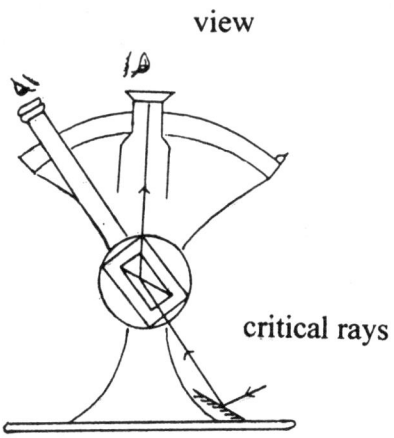

critical rays

Fig. 11..2. Abbe refractometer

EXERCISE NO. 11.2

To determine the effect of concentration on refrective index by Abbe refrectometer

Purpose

- To study the effect of concentration on the refractive index.

Requirements

Chemicals/reagents

- Sodium benzoate
- Sodium salicylate
- Or any substance
- Distilled water

Equipments/glasswares

Same as exercise 11.1

Procedure

1. Prepare stock solution of sodium benzoate of 1.0%.
2. Dilute the solution by aligation method till 0.1%, 0.2% ----------------0.9%
3. Determine refractive index of the given sample as exercise no. 11.1.
4. Determine density of substance at different concentration.

Observations

1. Experimental temperature   = t °C
2. Refractive index of water at t °C = ------

Table A. Density of test liquid

S.No.	Concentration (%)	Density of liquid
1.	1.0	
2.	2.0	
3.	3.0	
4.	4.0	
5.	5.0	
6.	6.0	
7.	7.0	
8.	8.0	
9.	9.0	
10.	1.0	

Table B. Refractive index

S.No.	Concentration (%)	Liquid			
		Refractive index			Mean
		(a)	(b)	(c)	
1.	0.1				
2.	0.2				
3.	0.3				
4.	0.4				
5.	0.5				
6.	0.6				
7.	0.7				
8	0.8				
9.	0.9				
10.	1.0				

Result

Plot the graph between concentration and refractive index and determine the concentration at which liquid shows highest refractive index.

EXERCISE NO. 11.3

To study the effect of temperature on refractive index by Abbe refrectometer.

Purpose

- To learn the effect of temperature on the refrective index when determined by Abbe refractometer.

Requirements

Chemicals/reagents

- Liquid or prepare one concentration of a substance.
- Distilled water

Equipments/glasswares

- Same as exercise no. 11.1

Procedure

1. Repeat the step 1 to 10 of exercise no. 11.1.
2. Increase the temperature and determine the refractive index of distilled water and test sample at the same temperature.
3. Determine density of liquid at different temperature using pycnometer or density bottle.
4. Plot the graph between temperature and refractive index.

Observations

1. Experimental temperature   = t °C
2. Refractive index of water at t °C = ------

Table A. Density of test liquid

S.No.	Temperature (°C)	Density of liquid
1.	Room temperature	
2.	37.5	
3.	45	
4.	55	

Tabe B Refractive index

Temperature (°C)	Distilled water				Liquid			
	Refractive index			Mean	Refractive index			Mean
	(a)	(b)	(c)		(a)	(b)	(c)	
1. 2. 3.								

Result

Plot the graph between temperature and refractive index and determine the temperature at which liquid shows highest refractive index.

Viva-voce Question Bank

1. What is refractive index?
2. How to determine refractive index?
3. What is index?
4. What is refractivity?
5. Why are you determine refrative index?
6. How factors effecting refractive index of substance?
7. Give princple Abbe refractometer.
8. Give method of determination of refractive index by Abbe refractometer.
9. What critical solution temperature?
10. Give principle of other apparatus which is used in the determination of refractive index

□□□

Chapter 12

CHEMICAL KINETICS

Chemical kinetics is a process related to various fundamentals of pharmaceutics from the manufacturer to the patient. It is essential to produce a stable, and non-toxic dosage form using fundamental conditions essential for the preparation of formulations. Kinetic principles have been applied in various field of pharmacy such as

(a) Stability of dosage form
(b) Incompatibility
(c) Dissolution study
(d) Pharmacokinetics
(e) Action of drug
(f) Other pharmaceutical factors

Rate of Reaction

The rate of a chemical reaction is defined as the velocity or speed of reaction at which a reactant or reaction undergo the chemical changes. The reactions which occur in single step are known as simple reaction or elementary reaction and those which take place in two or more steps are called as complex reaction. e.g.

$$A \longrightarrow Product \qquad\qquad --- (12.1)$$

a   0   initial concentration (t = 0)

a – x   x   after time t

$$Rate = \frac{moles\ of\ reactant\ used}{time\ required\ for\ this\ change} = \frac{x}{t} \qquad --- (12.2)$$

$$\text{Rate of reaction} = \pm (dc/dt)$$

In this expression (+) shows increase in the concentration while (−) shows decrease in concentration with a time interval dt.

Rate of reaction is directly proportional to the change in concentration.

$$dx / dt \propto (a - x) \qquad\qquad --- (12.3)$$
$$dx / dt = K (a - x) \qquad\qquad ---(12.4)$$

where, K is the rate constant or velocity constant or specific reaction rate. Unit of rate of reaction is mole litre^{-1}time^{-1}.

Factor Influencing Rate of Reaction

The rate of chemical reaction is represent in the term of reaction rate constant. The higher is the rate constant, faster is the reaction. The rate of reaction is affected by the the following parameters viz.

a. Internal factors

(a) pH (b) Ionic strength (c) Solvent (d) Catalyst
(e) Soluble gases (f) Other additives

b. External factors

(a) Temperature (b) Exposure of light (c) Radiation
(d) Moisture (e) Ambient air (f) Pressure

Factor Influencing Rate Constant

- Temperature
- Catalysts

Molecularity of Reaction

It is defined as the number of molecules of reactants taking part in a chemical reaction. It is a theoretical value and is derived from the mechanism of reaction. Molecularity can neither be zero nor fractional. Most of the reaction has molecularity less than 3. It is represented by the chemical reaction. e.g.

$$NH_4NO_3 \rightarrow N_2 + 2H_2O ; \qquad \text{molecularity} = 1$$
$$CH_3COOH + NaOH \rightarrow CH_3COONa + H_2O ; \qquad \text{molecularity} = 2$$
$$2NO + O_2 \rightarrow 2NO_2 \qquad\qquad \text{molecularity} = 3$$

Order of Reaction (OR)

It is defined as the number of molecules of reactants whose concentration determines the rate expression. It may be zero, integer or fractional. The order of reaction is the sum of the power of the concentration.

$$mA + nB \rightarrow product$$

According to law of mass of action

$$Rate = K[A]^m[B]^n$$

Order of reaction $= m + n$

$NH_4NO_3 \rightarrow N_2 + 2H_2O$;	$OR = m + n = 1 + 0 = 1$
$CH_3COOH + NaOH \rightarrow CH_3COONa + H_2O$;	$OR = m + n = 1 + 1 = 2$
$2NO + O_2 \rightarrow 2NO_2$;	$OR = m + n = 2 + 1 = 3$
$CH_3COOC_2H_5 + H_2O \rightarrow CH_3COOH + C_2H_5OH$;	$OR = m + n = 1 + 0 = 1$
$H_2 + Cl_2 \rightarrow 2HCl$;	$OR = m + n = 0 + 0 = 0$

Zero Order Reaction

A reaction is called to be zero order if the rate of reaction is independent on the concentration of the reactant e.g. photochemical reaction, enzymatic reaction etc.

$$A \leftrightarrow product \qquad -- (12.5)$$
$$a \qquad 0 \quad initially$$

> Reaction rate $dx / dt = K$ (constant)

First Order Reaction

A reaction is said to be first order if the concentration of one reactant is dependent is dependent on the concentration of the reactant and the rate of reaction is proportional to the first power of the concentration of the reaction. e.g.

$$A \leftrightarrow product \qquad --- (12.6)$$
$$a \qquad 0 \qquad initially$$
$$a - x \qquad x \qquad after \ time \ t$$

Rate of reaction $dx / dt \propto (a - x)$

$$dx / dt = K(a - x) \qquad --- (12.7)$$

where K is the reaction rate constant
after solving the equation (12.7)

$$K = \frac{2.303}{t} \log_{10} \frac{a}{a - x}$$

Second Order Reaction

A reaction is said to be of second order if the reaction velocity is directly proportional to the product of concentration of two substances. e.g.

Case I When reactant has same concentration

$$2A \leftrightarrow \text{product} \qquad\qquad \text{--- (12.8)}$$

a	0	initially
a – x	x	after time t

$$dx / dt \propto (a - x)^2 \qquad\qquad \text{--- (12.9)}$$

or

$$dx / dt = K(a - x)^2$$

after solving of this equation

$$\boxed{K = \frac{1}{t.a} \times \frac{x}{(a - x)}}$$

Case II When reactant have different concentrations

$$A + B \leftrightarrow \text{product} \qquad\qquad \text{--- (12.10)}$$

a	b	0	initially
a – x	b – x	2x	after time t

$$dx / dt \propto (a - x)(b - x) \qquad\qquad \text{--- (12.11)}$$

or

$$dx / dt = K(a - x)(b - x)$$

after solving this equation

$$\boxed{K = \frac{2.303}{t(a - b)} \log_{10} \frac{b(a - x)}{a(b - x)}}$$

Important facts about Order of Reactions

Order	Unit of K	Half life
Zero	mole litre^{-1}time^{-1}	$t_{1/2} = a / 2.K$
First	time^{-1}	$t_{1/2} = 0.693 / K$
Second	litre mole^{-1}time^{-1}	$t_{1/2} = 1 / K.a$
Third	litre^2 mole^{-2}time^{-1}	$t_{1/2} = 3 / 2K.a^2$

Determination of Order of Reaction

Following methods are commonly used for the determination of order of reaction

(a) Graphic method
(b) Substitution method
(c) Half life method
(d) Integration method or Hit and Trial method
(e) Vant't Hoff differential method

EXERCISE NO. 12.1

To determine the velocity constant of the hydrolysis of given compound.

Purpose

- To determine velocity constant of the hydrolysis of given compounds

Requirements

Chemicals/reagents

- Methyl acetate
- Hydrochloric acid
- Sodium hydroxide

Equipments/glasswares

- Thermostat
- Thermometer
- Conical flask

$$CH_3COOCH_3 + H_2O \longrightarrow CH_3COOH + CH_3OH$$

methy acetate   acetic acid   methanol

a   0   0   initially

a – x   x   x   after t time

velocity of reaction, $dx/dt = K[CH_3COOCH_3][H_2O]$ --- (12.12)

Procedure

1. Put methyl acetate and 0.5N HCl in thermostat for about 30 min in separate flask.
2. Maintain the temperature of thermostat.
3. Mix 15 ml of methyl acetate and 75 ml of 0.5N HCl at a particular temperature.
4. Take 5ml of sample immediately and titrate by standardized 0.1N NaOH solution using phenolphthalein as indicator.
5. Cool the container using cold water or add ice piece in the thermostat to freeze the equilibrium.
6. Repeat step 5 by withdrawing 5 ml of sample at a fix interval of time.
7. Take the samples till hydrolysis of ester is complete.
8. In the titration, the amount of NaOH required, is equal to the total of amount of HCl added and the amount of acetic acid generated in the chemical reaction.
9. The amount of acetic acid produced after a interval of time t can be estimated by titration.
10. Velocity of reaction and $t_{1/2}$ is calculated by applying mathematical equation.

Observations

(a) Temperature (at which study carried out) = ------°C
(b) Volume of HCl added = ---- ml
(c) Volume of methyl acetate taken = ----- ml

Observation table

S.No	Time (minute)	Volume of sample withdrawn (ml)	Burette reading Initial (a)	Burette reading Final (b)	Volume of NaOH required (b –a) ml
1	0	5			$= V_0$
2	10	5			
3	20	5			
4	30	5			
5	40	5			
6	50	5			
7	60	5			
-	-	5			
-	-	5			$= V_\infty$

Calculation

The amount of acetic acid formed at the completion of the reaction is equal to the initial amount, a of methyl acetate is hydrolyzed.

Let V_0, V_t and V_∞ be the volume of 0.1N NaOH solution required at zero, time t and infinite (∞) time respectively

(i) The amount of acetic acid (x) produced after time t $\propto V_t - V_0$
(ii) The initial concentration of methyl acetate (a) $\propto V_\infty - V_0$

Amount of ester present at time t, i.e.

$$(a - x) \propto (V_\infty - V_0) - (V_t - V_0)$$
$$(a - x) \propto V_\infty - V_t$$

The value of K is calculated by applying first order reaction e.g.

$$K = \frac{2.303}{t} \log_{10} \frac{V_\infty - V_0}{V_\infty - V_t}$$

The value of velocity constant can be calculated at different intervals of time and half life of the reaction is calculated by the following equation

$$t_{1/2} = 0.693 / K$$

Result

The velocity constant of the given reaction is ------ min^{-1} and half life period of the reaction is ----- min.

EXERCISE NO. 12.2

To determine the relative strength of two acids

Purpose

- To learn method of determination of relative strength of two acids.
- To study the hydrolysis of ester by acid.

Requirements

Chemicals/reagents

- Methyl acetate (CH_3COOCH_3)
- Hydrochloric acid (HCl)
- Sulphuric acid (H_2SO_4)
- Distilled water
- Sodium hydroxide (NaOH)
- Phenolphthalein indicator

Equipments/glasswares

- Thermostat
- Thermometer
- Conical flask
- Beaker (50 ml, 100 ml, and 250 ml)
- Pipette (10 ml)

$$CH_3COOCH_3 + H_2O \xrightarrow{\text{acid}} CH_3COOH + CH_3OH$$

methy acetate		acetic acid	methanol	
a		0	0	initially
a − x		x	x	after t time

velocity of reaction, $dx / dt = K[CH_3COOCH_3][H_2O]$ --- (12.13)

water is present in large excess hence,

$$dx / dt = K[CH_3COOCH_3] \qquad\qquad \text{--- (12.14)}$$

Procedure

1. Determine the rate constant of the hydrolysis of methyl acetate by 0.1N HCl at a definite temperature like room temperature or 30°C as Ex. 6.1.
2. Determine the rate constant of the hydrolysis of methyl acetate by 0.1N H_2SO_4 at a definite temperature like room temperature or 30°C as step 1.
3. Calculate rate constant applying first order reaction (K_1 and K_2).

Observations

(a) Temperature (at which study carried out) = ------°C
(b) Volume of HCl added = ---- ml
(c) Volume of H_2SO_4 added = ---- ml
(d) Volume of methyl acetate taken = ----- ml

Observation Table A (hydrolysis of ester by HCl)

S.No.	Time (minute)	Volume of sample withdrawn (ml)	Burette reading Initial (a)	Final (b)	Volume of NaOH required (b –a) ml
1	0	5			$= V_0$
2	10	5			
3	20	5			
-	-	-			$= V_\infty$

Observation Table B (hydrolysis of ester by H_2SO_4)

S.No.	Time (minute)	Volume of sample withdrawn (ml)	Burette reading Initial (a)	Final (b)	Volume of NaOH required (b –a) ml
1	0	5			$= V_0$
2	10	5			
3	20	5			
-	-	-			$= V_\infty$

Calculation

The relative strength of acids is determined by the following equation

$$\text{Relative strength} = \frac{\text{strength of one acid}}{\text{strength of other acid}} = \frac{\alpha_1}{\alpha_2} = \frac{K_1}{K_2} \qquad \text{--- (12.15)}$$

Result

The velocity constant of the given acids (HCl and H_2SO_4) are --- &--- min^{-1} respectively and relative strength of given acids is ------.

Precautions

1. Both flasks containing esters and acid should be heated at same temperature using thermostat.
2. First sample should be withdrawn immediately as quickly as possible.
3. Distilled water should be used throughout the study.
4. V_∞ is determined by the continuos sampling at which the titration value is constant.
5. Titration should be preformed carefully.
6. Repeat experiments two to three times till you get satisfied.

EXERCISE NO. 12.3

To determine the saponification value of given ester

Purpose

- To learn determination of saponification value of ethyl acetate by chemical kinetics.
- To familirise the student with saponification due to its importance in determining the HLB value of surfactant.

Requirements

Chemicals/reagents

- Ethyl acetate ($CH_3COOC_2H_5$)
- Hydrochloric acid (HCl)
- Sodium hydroxide (NaOH)
- Phenolphthalein indicator

Equipments/Glasswares

Same as exercise no. 12.2

Chemical reaction

$$CH_3COO\ C_2H_5 + NaOH \longrightarrow CH_3COONa + C_2H_5OH$$

ethyl acetate   acetic acid   methanol

velocity of reaction, $dx/dt = K[CH_3COOCH_3][NaOH]$ -- (12.16)

Procedure

1. Prepare 0.01M ethyl acetate in distilled water by dissolving 0.22 g of ethyl acetate in 250 ml of distilled water and if necessary filter it.
2. Prepare 0.02M NaOH and 0.02M HCl in distilled water each 500 ml in separate flask and label properly.
3. Take 50 ml of ester solution in 250 ml stoppered conical flask and 50 ml of sodium hydroxide solution in separate stoppered conical flask. Place both flask on the thermostat at 30°C for 30 min.
4. After maintaining the temperature of both flask, pour the alkali solution into ester solution and shake this flask thoroughly.
5. Start the stop watch immediately when two solutions are mixed.
6. Take 10 ml of sample at interval of 5,10, 15, -----min.
7. Withdrawn sample is to be discharged rapidly into the flask containing 10 ml of hydrochloric acid solution.
8. Titrate the excess of acid with standard alkali solution using phenolphthalein as an indicator.

9. Repeat the step 7 and 8 after withdrawing of sample at fix interval of time.
10. Calculate the initial concentration of alkali (a) and concentration of ester (b) by titration.
11. Allow the remaining mixture of alkali and ester for 24 h for the completion of reaction and determine the final volume of titre V_∞.

Observations

(a) Temperature = ---- °C
(b) Molecular weight of ethylacetate = 88
(c) Density of the ethylacetate = 0.9005

Table A. Standardization of solutions

Time (min.)	Volume of HCl	Burette reading		Volume of NaOH required(V_t)	$(a - x) = (V - V_t)$	$(b - x) = (V_\infty - V_t)$
		Initail	Final			
0.0				$V_0 =$		
30						
60						
90						
-						
-						
-						
∞				V_∞		

Calculation

Second order of the reaction, the constant calculated by the following reaction.

$$K = \frac{2.303}{t(a-b)} \log_{10} \frac{b(a-x)}{a(b-x)}$$

Where a and b are the initial concentration of alkali and ester.

$a \equiv (V - V_0)$ ml
$(a - x) \equiv$ amount of NaOH present at time t.
$\equiv$ amount of HCl used

$\equiv$ difference of the amount of acid present initially and the amount of acid present initially and the amount of acid present at time t.

$\equiv (V - V_t)$ ml

$x \equiv a - (a - x) \equiv (V_t - V_0)$ ml

$(a - b) \equiv$ excess of sodium hydroxide over ester

$\equiv$ unreacted amount of sodium hydroxide at the end of the reaction.

$\equiv (V - V_\infty)$

Hence constant b

$b = a - (a - x) \equiv (V_\infty - V_0)$

and

$(b - x) = (V_\infty - V_0) - (V_t - V_0) \equiv (V_\infty - V_t)$

Calculation value of K by the following equation,

$$K = \frac{2.303}{t\,(a - b)} \log_{10} \frac{b\,(a - x)}{a\,(b - x}$$

Result

The order of saponification of ethyl acetate = ----.

EXPERIMENT NO. 12.4

To investigate the reaction between acetone and iodine

Purpose

- To study the reaction between acetone and iodine and leaen how to determine order of the reaction.

Requirements

Chemicals/reagents

- Acetone
- Iodine
- Acid

Equipments/glasswares

- Burette
- Burette stand
- Thermostat
- Beaker & conical flask
- Pipette

Procedure

1. Take acetone, iodine solution and acid in a thermostat for about 45 min.
2. Prepare different concentration of solutions in four different bottle and place the level properly.
3. Mix the solution homogeneously for a few min.
4. Take 10 ml of this solution from one bottle in separate conical flask.
5. Add 10 ml N-sodium acetate solution for identification of reaction.
6. Analyse the sample by titration using N/100 sodium thiosulphate as titrant in the solution and employed starch solution as an indicator.
7. Take sample after a fix interval of time and analyse it in the same way as discussed above.
8. Proceed the exeperiment in the same way for all three composition.
9. The titrate values are taken proportional to the iodine concentration.
10. Repeat the exercise for accuracy and for concept of the chemical reaction.

Observations

Observation table for composition of solutions

S.No.	Container	Acetone (ml)	0.5 N Sulphuric acid (ml)	0.1N Iodine solution (ml)	Distilled water (ml)
1.	A	5	25	10	70
2.	B	7.5	22.5	12.5	66.5
3.	C	10	20	15	55
4.	D	10	25	7.5	57.5

Observation for reaction

S.No.	Containet A		Container B		Container C		Container D	
	Time (min.)	Volume of sol. (ml)	Time (min.)	Volume of sol. (ml)	Time (min.)	Volume of sol. (ml)	Time (min.)	Volume of sol. (ml)
1.	10							
2.	20							
3.	30							
4.	40							

Calculation

Plot a graph between time value of the titre and find out slope of the each concentration of the solution. Velocity constant of the reaction is determine by the slope of graph.

Result

The reaction follows -----------order of the reaction and velosity constant of the reaction -----------.

Viva-voce Question Bank

(A) Short answer type question
1. What is chemical kinetics?
2. What is order of reaction?
3. What is molecularity?
4. How to differentiate order of reaction and molecularity of reaction?
5. What is rate constant?
6. How many factors affecting order of reaction?
7. Why are you determining order of reaction?
8. Give three examples of zero order of reaction.
9. What is pseudo first order reaction?
10. How to determine first order rate constant?
11. What is kinetics?
12. How to determine half life of reaction?
13. How to determine shelf life?
14. What is $t_{20\%}$?
15. Give equation of first order of reaction.
16. What is importance of chemical kinetics in pharmacy?
17. What is the role kinetics in the formulation of dosage forms?
18. What is law of mass action?
19. How to determine temperature coefficient?
20. What is unit of rate constant of first order reaction?

(B) State true/false
1. The unit of rate of reaction changes with the changes of order of reaction.
2. Rate of reaction depends upon surface area of reactants.
3. All radioactive decays obey zero order reaction.
4. The rate an endothermic reaction increases with decreasing temperature.
5. All zero order reactions are unimlecular.
6. Time required to complete half of the reactant in a zero order reaction is equal to 1/2K.
7. The rate constant of most the ionic reactions do not decreases with increase in temperature.
8. All zero order reactions are bimolecular.
9. The rate of reaction decreases with time
10. Molecularity of reaction is never in fractional.

Answer(B) State true/false
      1.F   2.T   3.F   4.F   5.F   6.F   7.F   8.F   9.T   10.T

❏❏❏

MICROMERITICS

Micromeritics involves the study of small particles in micron size. The control of size and the size range of particles play an important role in pharmacy. Following characteristics of particles are studied under the micromeritics.

(a) Size (b) Shape (c) Volume (d) Density

(e) Surface area (f) Flow properties (g) Porosity

The study of particle size and particle size distribution plays has importance in pharmacy. It is useful particularly in studying.

1. Physical properties of power & flow characteristic of power
2. Release and dissolution control
3. Solubility of substances
4. Rate of absorption & stability of pharmaceutical products
5. Uniformity of dose
6. Mixing of powder
7. Filtration & centrifugation
8. Elegance of products

Table 13.1. Particle dimension in disperse system

S.No.	Particle size (μm)	Approximate sieve size	Example
1.	0.5-10	-	Suspension, fine emulsion
2.	10 – 50	-	Coarse emulsion, flocculated suspension
3.	50 –100	325>140	Fine particles
4.	150 – 1000	100>180	Coarse power
5.	1000 - 3360	18>6	Average granule size

Table 13.2. Standards of sieve

S.No.	Sieve no.	Opening size (μm)	Opening size (mm)	Permissible variation in maximum opening (%)	Diameter of wire(mm)
1.	02	9520	9.5200	+05	2.110 – 2.590
2.	04	4760	4.7600	+10	1.140 – 1.680
3.	08	2380	2.3800	+10	0.740 – 1.100
4.	10	2000	2.0000	+10	0.680 – 1.000
5.	20	0840	0.8400	+15	0.380 – 0.550
6.	30	0590	0.5900	+15	0.290 – 0.420
7.	40	0420	0.4200	+25	0.230 – 0.330
8.	50	0297	0.2970	+25	0.170 – 0.253
9.	60	0250	0.2500	+25	0.149 – 0.220
10.	70	0210	0.2100	+25	0.130 – 0.187
11.	80	0177	0.1770	+40	0.114 – 0.154
12.	100	0149	0.1490	+40	0.096 – 0.125
13.	120	0125	0.1250	+40	0.079 – 0.103
14.	200	0074	0.0740	+60	0.045 – 0.061

Particle Size and Size Distribution

The size of a sphere is generally expressed in terms of its diameter though it is generally asymmetric in nature. The size of particles can be expressed as

(a) Surface diameter (ds)
(b) Volume diameter (dp)
(c) Projected diameter (dst)
(d) Sieve diameter (dsieve)
(e) Volume-surface diameter (dvs)

If particle is spherical in nature, the surface area can be determined by

$$S = \pi d^2$$

and,   volume of particles (V) = $\dfrac{\pi d^3}{6}$

But most of powders are non-spherical. Hence, it is not possible to express its size in terms of its diameter. The size of non-spherical particles can be expressed in term of equivalent spherical diameters and can be expressed as

Surface diameter (ds) : Diameter of a sphere which have the same surface area as that of the asymmetric particles.

Volume diameter (dv) : Diameter of a sphere which have same volume as that of the asymmetric particles.

Projected diameter (dp) : Diameter of a sphere which have the same area of asymmetric particles when obsered under the microscope.

Stoke's diameter (dst) : Diameter of an equivalent sphere undergoing sedimentation at the same rate as the asymmetric particles.

Sieve diameter (dsieve) : Ddiameter of a sphere that passes through the same sieve aperature as the asymmetric particle.

Characterization of Powder Size

Powder is considered as group of small particles. Most of powders contain more than one size of particles are known as polydisperse if powder contains one size of particles is called as monodisperse. There is no universal method for determining the size of power but in pharmacy it can be descrived in the form of arithmetic means and some times it is applicable in the form of geometric and haemonic means.

Arithmetic mean of a powder is defined as the geometrical sum of the various particle sizes divided by the number of particles. General equation for the average particle size may be in any mean diameter like arithmetic, geometric or harmonic means

$$d_{mean} = \frac{(\Sigma nd^{p+f})^{1/p}}{(\Sigma nd)^{1/p}}$$

where n is the number of particle in size range whose midpoint. P is an index related to the size of an individual particles and f is the frequency index.

Table 13.3. Statistical arithmetic mean diameter of powders

S.No.	p	f	Equation	Size number	Frequency	Mean diameter
1	1	0	$\Sigma nd/\Sigma n$	Length	Number	Length number mean (d_{ln})
2	2	0	$(\Sigma nd/\Sigma n)^{1/2}$	Surface	Number	Surface number mean (d_{sn})
3	3	0	$(\Sigma nd/\Sigma n)^{1/3}$	Volume	Number	Volume number mean (d_{vn})
4	1	1	$\Sigma nd^2/\Sigma nd$	Length	Length	Surface length mean (d_{sl})
5	1	2	$\Sigma nd^3/\Sigma nd^2$	Length	Surface	Volume surface mean (d_{vs})
6	1	3	$\Sigma nd^4/\Sigma nd^3$	Length	Weight	Weight moment mean(d_{wm})

Determination of Particle Size

Following methods are generally employed for the determination of particle size and particle size distribution.

1. Microscopic method

Microscopic method is generally employed for measurement of particle size in the range of 0.2 – 100 μm. For accuracy and good estimation of particle size distribution about 300 – 500 particles must be counted. In this method, the size of particle is represented in the form of projected diameter. This method is suitable to estimate particle size of suspension and globule size of emulsions.

Advantages of microscopic method

1. Easy to see the view of the particles.
2. Agglomeration of particles can be detected using this techniques.
3. Simple and accurate method within a certain limit of the particle size.

Disadvantages of microscopic method

1. Only length and width of particles can be measured by this method. Depth of the particle can not be measured by this method.
2. Time consuming methods, as it required to count more than 500 particle for accuracy.

2. Sieving method

This method is most suitable to determine the particle size of powder range between 50 – 1500 μm. In this method, the powder is placed on the set of sieve in which the sieves arranged in gradually decreasing order of pore size. This set of sieves are shake for a definite period using a mechanical shaker. Material which is retained on each sieve is collected and weighed. Size is expressed in the form of dsieve which descrives the diameter of a sphere that passes through the sieves aperture. Sieve which are employed in pharmaceutical testing are constructed from wire cloth with square meshes, woven from wire of brass, bronze, stainless steel or any other material which can not react with material and helpful in the sieving of the substances

Advantages
1. It exhibits reproducible results.
2. It is economic.
3. The method is very suitable for the determination of the power size

Disadvantages
1. It is not suitable for powder having particle size less than 50 μm..
2. Moisture some times create problem for the determination of the particle size.

Table 13.4. IP Specification of sieves

S.No.	Sieve number	Aperture size (μm)	S.No.	Sieve number	Aperture size (μm)
1.	10	1700	8.	44	325
2.	12	1400	9.	60	250
3.	16	1000	10.	85	35
4.	22	710	11.	100	-
5.	25	600	12.	120	-
6.	30	500	13.	150	-

3. Sedimentation method

The rate of settling of particles in a suspension or emulsion may be determined by Stoke's law and it is determined by the following equation known as Stoke's equation

$$dst = \sqrt{\frac{18\eta_0 h}{(\rho_s - \rho_0)gt}}$$

where, h is the distance of fall of particles in time t sec, η_0 is the viscosity of medium in cps, ρ_s is the density of the particles, ρ_0 is the density of the dispersion medium and g is the acceleration due to gravity.

4. Conductivity method

Particle size ranging from 0.5 μm to 500 μm is determined by conductivity method. In this method, volume of particle is measured and changed into diameter of particles. Coulter counter apparatus is employed for the determination of particle volume. Principle of this instrument is based on particle suspended in a conducting liquid passes through a small orifice on either side of electrode and alteration of the electric resistance. For determination of particle size of suspension a known volume of dilute suspension is pumped through the orifice and a constant voltage is applied across the electrodes, it produce a current. When particles passes through the orifice it displaces its own volume of the electrolyte due to this change resistance between the two electrodes is increased. The change of resistance is related to the particle volume and pulses height analyzer calibrated in terms of particle size.

Particle Size Distribution

Particle size distribution can be expressed in two ways

1. Determining the number of particles present in each size range and represented by frequency distribution curve and cumulative frequency plot. It can be determined by microscopic techniques.
2. Determining the weight of particles present in each size range and determining by sedimentation and sieving method.

EXERCISE NO. 13.1

To determine the particle size distribution of powder by sieving method

Purpose

- To learn the method for determining particle size distribution.
- To learn handling of sieve and factors affecting the particle of size distribution.

In this techniques, particles of a powder substance are placed on the screen which have uniform apertures. When this sieve set is shaked using electrical instrument, the smaller particles than apertures are passed through the screen and higher particles are retained on the screen. The sieve motion is mainly of two types.

(a) Horizontal motion : By this type of motion particles tend to loosen the packing in contact with the surface screen and smaller particles are passed through the screen.

(b) Vertical motion : By this type of motion particles agitate are thoroughly mixed increasing the rate of sieving.

Industrial-size mechanical sieves are available in various design and capacity which includes various type of motion like gyratory, circular rotatory, vibrating, shaking, and revolving shifters.

Requirements

Chemicals/reagents

- Calcium carbonate/aspirin/calmine powder/any power substances

Equipments/Glasswares

- Sieve set (sieve no.30, 45, 60, 80, 100, 140, and 200)
- Electromagnetic laboratory sieve machine
- or electrical sieve shaker

Procedure

1. Arrange set of sieves in the descending order.
2. Weighed amount of sample is tube placed in the sieve at the top of the sieve set.
3. Start the sieving machine. The length of time and speed of vibration can be controlled by semiautomatic or automatic attachment in the machine.
4. Collect the powder material retained on the various sieves.
5. Weigh the powdered material retained on the sieve.
6. Calculate percent frequency of each size of particle and plot the graphs.
7. Determine the geometric mean weight diameter and geometrical standard deviation.

Observations

(a) Weight of substance $\quad$ = W_1 g
(b) Time of shaking $\quad$ = t $\quad$ min.
(c) Speed of electrical shaker $\quad$ = P $\quad$ rpm

Observation table

S.No.	Sieve number (passed/retained)	Arithmetic mean size of opening (μm)	Weight retained on a sieve (g)	Percent weight retained (undersize)	Cumulative percent retained
1	30/45	470			
2	45/60	300			
3	60/80	213			
4	80/100	163			
5	100/140	127			
6	140/200	90			

Calculation

Calculation of percent weight retained on screen

$$\text{Percent weight retained on screen} = \frac{\text{weight retained on screen}}{\text{Total weight of powder}} \times 100$$

1. Plot frequency distribution curve taking particle size on X axis and percent weight retained on the screen on Y axis.
2. The logarithm of the particle size is plotted against the cumulative percent frequency on a probability scale. It showed a linear relationship. The slope of the line and a reference point can be determined.
3. The geometrical mean weight diameter d_g and geometric standard deviation σ_g can be obtained form the straight line.

Following statistical diameters are calculated from weight distribution
(a) Length-number mean (d_{ln}) $\qquad$ $\log d_{ln} = \log d_g - 5.757 \log^2 \sigma_g$
(b) Suraface- number mean (d_{sn}) $\qquad$ $\log d_{sn} = \log d_g - 4.606 \log^2 \sigma_g$
(c) Volume- number mean (d_{vn}) $\qquad$ $\log d_{vn} = \log d_g - 3.454 \log^2 \sigma_g$
(d) Volume-surface mean $\quad$ (d_{vs}) $\qquad$ $\log d_{vs} = \log d_g - 1.151 \log^2 \sigma_g$
(e) Weight-moment mean $\quad$ (d_{wm}) $\qquad$ $\log d_{wm} = \log d_g + 3.454 \log^2 \sigma_g$

Result

The geometrical mean weight diameter d_g is -- & geometric standard dev.σ_g is ------- .

EXERCISE NO. 13.2

To determine particle size in disperse medium by microscopic method

Purpose

- To learn the principle and microsopic method for analysis of particle size in suspension and globules size in emulsion.
- To study the agglomeration of particles and to measure any contamination gross in the green sample of powder.

Requirements

Chemicals/reagents
- Paracetamol suspension
- Or disperse silica in water
- Distilled water

Equipments/glasswares

- Microscope
- Stage micrometer
- Oculometer
- Plain slides
- Pipette

Procedure

1. To prepare suspension of paracetamol by dispersing drug in aquous phase without dilution or take any powder and disperse in the purified water.
2. Clean the microscope and place it in proper place where light is suitable for projection.
3. Fix the eye-piece in microscope with micrometer.
4. Calibrate the eye-piece micrometer with a standard stage micrometer.
5. Take the powder and disperse it in aqueous phase or in liquid paraffin or use prepared suspension in dilute form.
6. Mount the sample on the plain slide.
7. Measure the size of the particles with the help of eye-piece micrometer.
8. Count accurately at least 300-500 particles.

Observations

(a) 1 division of stage micrometer $= 0.1$ mm

(b) N_1 division of eye-piece (oculometer) $\equiv N_2$ division of stage micrometer

Observation table

Size range in μm	Mean of size range	Mean of size range × least count (d) in μm	Number of particles (n)	Percent freque-ncy	nd	nd^2	nd^3	nd^4
1 –3	2							
3 – 5	4							
5 – 7	6							
7 – 9	8							
9 – 11	10							
11 – 13	12							
13 – 15	14							
15 – 17	16							
17 – 19	18							
19 – 21	20							
			$\Sigma n =$		$\Sigma nd =$	$\Sigma nd^2 =$	$\Sigma nd^3 =$	$\Sigma nd^4 =$

Calculation

(a) Least count of eye-piece $= \dfrac{N_2}{N_1} \times 0.1$ mm

(b) Arithmatic mean $= \Sigma nd / \Sigma n$

(c) Volume-surface mean diameter $= \Sigma nd^3 / \Sigma nd^2$

(d) Weight-moment mean diameter $= \Sigma nd^4 / \Sigma nd^3$

Result

- The arithmetic mean diameter of given powder is ----- μm, volume-surface mean diameter is ------- μm and weight-moment mean diameter is ----μm.
- Plot the
  (i)   Size frequency distribution curve
  (ii) log-normal
  (iii) cumulative frequency and
  (iv) probability curves.

EXERCISE NO. 13.3

To determine the globule size of emulsion by microscopic method

Purpose

- To learn the method of globules size determination in emulsion using microscopic method.
- To study the agglomeration of globules and other physical properties of globules.

Requirements

Chemicals/reagents
- Liquid paraffin
- or any other emulsion
- castor oil

Equipments/glasswares

- Microscope
- Stage micrometer
- Oculometer
- Plain slides
- Pipette

Procedure

Follow same procedure as in exercise no. 15.2.

Observations

Same as in exercise no. 15.2

Calculation

Same as in exercise no. 15.2

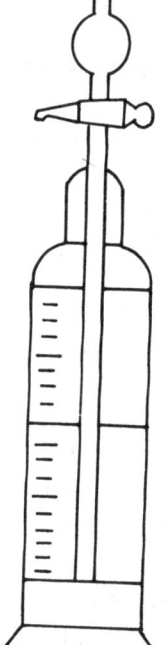

Fig. 13.1. Andreasen apparatus

Result

The globule mean diameter of emulsion is ------ μm.

Note : Sample of powders may be given for the determination of the true density occasionally combination of two material (one having slightly higher true density than the other) so that one can check the reliability of the result.

EXERCISE NO. 13.4

To determine particle size of dispersed medium by sedimentation method

Purpose

- To study the effect of gravity on sedimentation of particle size.
- To learn method of determination of particle size of powder.

Requirements

Chemicals/reagents

- Powder substance like kaolin, calcium carbonate, magnisium carbonate, etc
- Distilled water

Equipments/glasswares

- Andreasen apparatus
- Beaker
- Conical flask
- Petri dishes
- Oven

Procedure

1. Prepare slurry of the given powder material (1 to 2 percent in suitable medium).
2. If necessary, add deflocculating agent in suspension.
3. Fill the suspension in the Andreasen vessel of capacity 550 ml.
4. Place the stopper and shake the apparatus for uniform distribution of the particles in the suspension.
5. After uniform distribution of suspension remove the stopper and fix the two-way pipette and put the system at room temperature without disturbing the arrangement.
6. At a fixed interval 10 ml samples are to be withdrawn by the pipette and collect the suspension in watch glass or petri plate.
7. Remove the solvent from the samples by the evaporation till a constant weight is obtined.
8. Take weight of particles for each time interval. This weight is referred as weight undersize of particles.
9. This values are then converted in cumulative weight undersize.
10. Particle diameter is measured by Stoke's law.

Observations

(a) Concentration of powder suspension = percent
(b) Density of dispersed phase = g/cm³
(c) Density of dispersion medium = g/cm³
(d) Viscosity of suspension = cps

Observation table A

S.No.	Time interval (sec.)	Height of the suspension (cm)	Weight of power after drying (g)	Percent weight cf power (g)	Cumulative percent of powder weight
1.					
2.					
3.					
4.					
5.					
6.					
7.					
8.					
9.					
10.					

Calculation

Settling of particles in a suspension or globules in emulsion can be determined by the Stoke's equation.

$$d_{st} = [18\eta_0 h / (\rho_s - \rho_0)gt]^{1/2}$$

In this equation viscosity (η_0) of suspension is determined by Ostwald viscometer as discussed in exercise no.------------- and density of powder is determined as exercise no.-------.Density of medium is estimated as per the procedure mentioned in exercise---. Calculate the particle by taking average particles size.

Result

The average mean Stoke's diameter of particles is ------µm.

EXERCISE NO. 13.5

To determine surface area of the particles by permeability method

Purpose

• To learn principle of air permeability method and its importance.

Requirements

Chemicals/reagents

• Powder materials

Equipments/glasswares

• Fisher subsieve sizer apparatus
• Manometer

Procedure

1. Arrange the instrument properly.
2. Packed the power sample in the sample tube.
3. Connecte one end of the powder to an air pump through a constant pressure regulator while other end of the tube is connected to a calibrated manometer which contains suitable solvent of low viscosity and negligible vapor pressure.
4. Attach air pressure and maintain constant pressure regulator.
5. Moisture is removed by passing the dry air.
6. Pass the air through the packed powder in the sample tube.
7. Flow of air is measured by the manometer.
8. The change in the level of the fluid in the manometer is shows the average diameter of the particles.
9. Average particle diameter can be read from the chart supplied with the instrument.

Observations

(a) Cross sectional area of the bed (pack) $A =$ cm^2
(b) Volume of air passes through the bed $V =$ cm^3
(c) Viscosity of the air $\eta =$ cps
(d) Length of the sample tube $l =$ cm
(e) Time flow of air $t =$ sec.
(f) Constant $K = 5 \pm 0.5$
(g) Porosity of powder $\varepsilon =$ ---
(h) Pressure difference of the bed $\Delta P =$ ---- (manometer reading)
(i) Surface area per gram of powder $S_w = ?$ cm^2/g

Calculation

$$V = (A/\eta S_w^2) \times (\Delta P\, t/ Kl) \times \{\varepsilon/(1 - \varepsilon)^2\}$$

Result

The surface area of given power is ----- cm^2 and diameter of the powder is ----- μm.

EXERCISE NO. 13.6

To determine the true density of given powder by solvent displacement method

Purpose

- To learn the utility of density in the pharmacy.
- To learn the method of determination of true density of the given powder sample.

Requirements

Chemicals/reagents
- Powder substance like chalk /lactose/ magnesium carbonate/zinc oxide
- Solvent (benzene or any other solvent in which powder is insoluble)

Equipments/glasswares

Same as exercise no 13.2 &13.5

Procedure

1. Take weight of clean and dry density bottle.
2. Take weight of density bottle with small quantity of powder substance.
3. Now fill the density bottle by solvent without removing the powder material.
4. Take further weight of the density bottle, powder with the solvent.
5. Repeat the step 3 to 5 and take average.
6. Calculate the true density of the given power sample.
7. For reproducible results take all precaution as necessary.

Observations
(a) Weight of density bottle $= W_1$ g
(b) Weight of density bottle and powder sample $= W_2$ g
(c) Weight of density bottle + powder sample + solvent $= W_3$ g

Calculation

Weight of powder sample $= W_2 - W_1$
True volume occupied by the powder $= W_3 - W_2$

$$\boxed{\text{True density} = \text{weight of power} / \text{true volume of powder}}$$

$$\text{True density } (\rho) = (W_2 - W_1)/ (W_3 - W_2)$$

Result
True density of the given powder sample(s) is /are -----and -----.

EXERCISE NO. 13.7

To determine the true density of given powder by compressed powder method

Purpose

- To learn removal of space inside the powder.
- To study the effect of void space inside the powder.
- To study the methods and their importance in the removal of spaces.

Requirements

Chemicals/reagents
- Powder substances

Equipments/glasswares

- Tablet punching machine
- Hardness tester/Vernier calipers/Electrical balance

Procedure

1. Take powder material and pass through a suitable sieve size.
2. Compress the powder material using comperession force about to 1,00,000 lb/sq.inch.
3. Prepare at least 20 tablets by this compression techniques.
4. Select 10 tablet out of 20 which uniformity and have no any breakage problem.
5. Take weight of individual tablets
6. Measure the volume of individual tablet using caliperse.

Observations

Observation table

S.No.	Wt.of ind. tablet	Average weight of tablet (W)	Radius of tablet	Thickness of tablet	Volume of tablet	Av.volume of tab.(V)
1.						
2.						
3.						
4.						

Calculation

True density = weight of the tablet/volume of tablet

Result
True density of the given power material = --------g/cm^3

XERCISE NO. 13.8

To determine the bulk density of the given powder

Purpose

- To learn the method of determination of the bulk density.
- To learn the importance of bulk density in the field of pharmacy

Requirements

Chemicals/reagents

- Lactose /talc/other powdered materials

Equipments/Glasswares

Bulk density apparatus

Procedure

1. Take about 70 g of powder and pass through sieve no. 20.
2. Accurately weigh about 50 g.
3. Fill the powder in a 100 ml capacity measuring cylinder .
4. Fix the measuring cylinder on the bulk density apparatus.
5. Start the apparatus and control the tapping by the timer attached with a the instrument.
6. Not ethe bulk volume after tapping.
7. Or the bulk volume is determined by dropping the cylinder on the wooden surface three time height about 1 inch for 2 minutes

Observations

(a) Weight of powder   = m
(b) Bulk volume of power   = V
(c) Number of tapping   = ----
(d) Room temperature   =-------

Calculation

Bulk density = mass of powder / bulk volume of powder

Result

The bulk density of the powder = ----- g/cm^3

XERCISE NO. 13.9

To determine the granular density of given sample

Purpose

- To learn the utility of granule density in the manufacturing of tablets.
- To learn the method of determination of granule density.

Requirements

Chemicals/reagents

- Granules/powder
- Mercury

Equipments/glasswares

- Density bottle
- Beaker
- Glass funnel
- Electrical balance

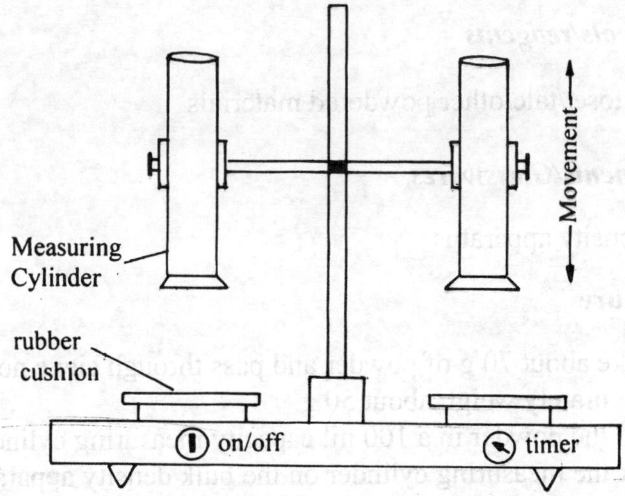

Measuring Cylinder

rubber cushion

on/off   timer

Fig. 11.2. Bulk density apparatus

Procedure

1. Take weight of clean and dry density bottle.
2. Take weight of density bottle and mercury
3. Take weight of density bottle with small quantity of granules.
4. Now fill the density bottle mercury without removing the granules.
5. Take further weight of the density bottle, granules with the mercury.
6. Repeat the step 3 to 5 and take average.
7. Calculate the granules density .
8. For reproducible results take all precaution as necessary.

Observations

Same as exercise no. 13.5

Calculation

Granule density = weight of granules/granules volume

Result

Granules density of the given powder sample(s) is /are ------ and -----.

EXERCISE NO. 13.10

To determine porosity, intra-particle porosity, interspace or void porosity and total porosity of powder

Purpose

- To learn the importance of void volume in packaging as well stability.

Requirements

Chemicals/reagents

Same as exercise no. 13.5 and 13.7

Equipments/glasswares

Same as exercise no. 13.5 and 13.7

Observations

Same as exercise no. 13.5 and 13.7

Calculations

(a) Porosity = (bulk volume – true volume)/ bulk volume
(b) Porosity = (true density – bulk density)/ true density
(c) Intra-particle porosity = (granule volume – true volume)/ granule volume
(d) Intra-particle volume = granule volume – true volume
(e) Interspace volume = bulk volume – granule volume
(f) Interspace porosity = (bulk volume – granule volume)/ bulk volume
(g) Total porosity = (true density – bulk density)/ true density
(h)

For determination of the parameter follows exercise no. 13.6, 13.7, and 13.8

Result

The porosity of the given material = -----, intraparticle volume = ----- and interspace volume = --------------.

EXERCISE NO. 13.11

To determine the angle of repose of the given powder material

Purpose

- To study flow property of powder and its importance in the field of pharmacy.

Requirements

Chemicals/reagents
Powder materials

Equipments/glasswares

Angle of repose apparatus/funnel/burette stand

Procedure

1. Place a glass funnel on a ring supported by a stand.
2. Take 50 g of powder sample and pass through sieve no. 20.
3. Block the orifice of the funnel by thumb.
4. Fill the powder in the funnel and remove the thunb immediately.
5. Maintain the gap between the bottom of the funnel and the top of the powder pile.
6. After emptying the powder from the funnel, measure the height of the pile and diameter.

Observations

(a) Temperature $= t\ °C$
(b) Weight of the power $=$ -----
(c) Sieve size used $=$ -------

Observation table

Glid-ant.	Conc.of glidant	Height of pile			Average hieght	Diameter of the pile			Average diameter
		(i)	(ii)	mean		(i)	(ii)	mean	

Calculation

Calculate the angle of repose, $\tan θ = 2h/ D = h/ r$

Result

The angle of repose of the given powders $=$-----, ------, ------and -----(Plot graph also).

EXERCISE NO. 13.12

To study the effect glidant on flow properties of powder

Purpose

- To study flow property of powder and its importance in the field of pharmacy.

Requirements

Chemicals/reagents

- Powder materials
- Glidants

Equipments/glasswares

Angle of repose apparatus/funnel/burette stand

Procedure

1. Place a glass funnel on a ring supported by a stand.
2. Take 50 g of powder sample and pass through sieve no. 20.
3. Block the orifice of the funnel by thumb.
4. Fill the powder in the funnel and remove the thunb immediately.
5. Add glidants in different ratios and perform same as exercise no. 13.11.
6. Maintain the gap between the bottom of the funnel and the top of the powder pile.
7. After emptying the powder from the funnel, measure the height of the pile and diameter.

Observations

    (d) Temperature   = t °C
    (e) Weight of the power = -----
    (f) Sieve size used   = -------

Observation table

Glid-ant.	Conc.of glidant	Height of pile			Average hieght	Diameter of the pile			Average diameter
		(i)	(ii)	mean		(i)	(ii)	mean	

Calculation

      Calculate the angle of repose, $\tan \theta = 2h/D = h/r$

Result

    The angle of repose of the given powders =-----, ------, ------and -----. The flow property of substance increases/decreases with inceasing of amount of glidants. (Plot graph also).

EXERCISE NO. 13.13

To determine compressibility index of power

Purpose

- To learn the method of determination of the compressibility index and its importance in the dosage form.

Requirements

Chemicals/reagents

Powder substance

Equipments/glasswares

Measuring cylinder
Spatula
Butter paper
Glass funnel

Procedure

1. Take measuring cylinder of capacity 10 ml.
2. Place the measuring cylinder on a plane surface.
3. Powder substance pass through sieve (no. 20) before use
4. Weigh amount of power is added carefully using the glass funnel or using paper without washing materials.
5. Measure the volume of the powder, called as fluffy volume.
6. Tap the measuring cylinder using tapping apparatus or on the wooden surface or on the pad.
7. Record the volume obtained after 50 tapping for 50 times.
8. If you want to knowing the effect of tapping , record the volume after a fix tapping (volume of the powder after 5, 10, 15 ---- 50 tapping).
9. Compressibility index is determined in percent.

Observations

(a) Temperature (room temperature) $= t \,°C$
(b) Weight of power $= W_g$
(c) Initial volume of the powder (fluffy volume) $= V_0$
(d) Volume of the powder after 50 taping 50 times $= V_t$

Table A. Measuring of volume after tapping

S.No.	Number of tapping	Volume of powder
1.	00	V_0
2.	10	
3.	15	
4.	20	
5.	25	
6.	30	
7.	40	
8.	50	V_t

Calculation

(a) Fluffy density of powder $= W/V_0$
(b) Tapped density $\quad\quad = W/V_t$

Compressibility index of the liquid is determined by the following equation.

$$\text{Compressibility Index (\%)} = \frac{\text{tapped density} - \text{fluffy density}}{\text{tapped density}} \times 100$$

Result

Compressibility of the given power material after 50 tapping = -----%.

EXERCISE NO. 13.14

To determine dispersibility of powder using hollow cylindrical method

Purpose

- To learn the utility and method of determination of the dispersibility of the powder material during the manufacturing.

Requirements

Chemicals/reagents

Same or different powder material as taken in exercise no. 13.12.

Equipments/glasswares

- Hollow cylinder
- Watch glass
- Balance

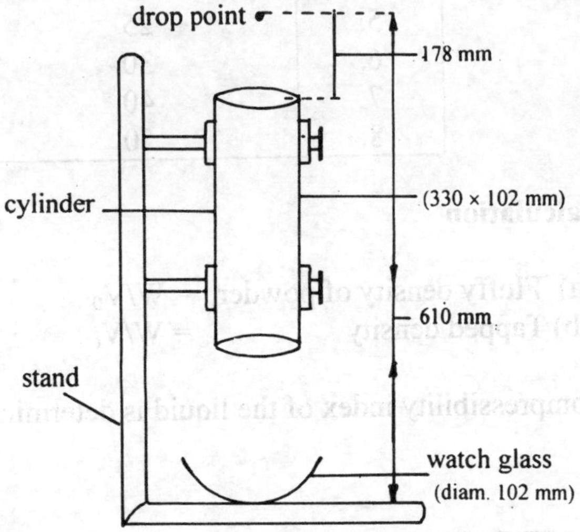

Procedure

1. Take weighed amount of powder (10 g).
2. Dispersibility apparatus should be fixed in stand, so that it can not be disturbed during the practical.
3. Drop the power material carefully from a fixed height as per the specification of the instrument.
4. Weigh powder material collected on the watch glass (diameter 120 mm).
5. Calculate the dispersibility in percent.

Fig. 11.3. Dispersibility apparatus

Observations

(a) Temperature (room temperature) = t °C
(b) Weight of powder = W g.
(c) Weight on watch glass = M

Calculation

$$\text{Dispersibility (\%)} = \frac{\text{Weight of powder on the watch glass}}{\text{Initial weight of the power}} \times 100$$

Result

Dispersibilty of the power = ----%.

Viva-voce Question Bank

(A) Short answer type question

1. What is micromeritics?
2. What is true density, granule density and bulk density?
3. What is porosity? explain with examples.
4. Give methods for determination of particle size.
5. What are the advantages and disadvantages of microscopic method used for the determination of particle size?
6. What is the principles of coulter counter and its principles.
7. What is specific surface of particles?
8. What is derived properties of powder?
9. Describe various methods of quantifying the flow properties of powder.
10. How to determine porosity of powder?
11. Define contact angle.
12. What is angle of repose. How it is useful in the pharmacy?
13. Give factors affecting dissolution rate of drug. What is the role of particle size distribution in the formulation?
14. Give advantages and disadvantages of sedimentation method used for determination of the particle size.
15. Give importance of particle size distribution in the manufacturing of tablet and capsule.
16. How will you determine the particle distribution of powder?
17. What is the role of bulkiness and compressibility of powder in the manufacturing of the dosage forms.
18. What is void volume?

(B) Define the following terms with examples.

(a) Angle of repose
(b) Porosity
(c) Derived property of power
(d) Contact angle
(e) Bulkiness
(f) Dustibility
(g) Stoke's law
(h) Coulter counter
(i) Bulk density
(j) Granule density
(k) Lubricant and glidant
(l) Surface texture
(m) Sieving method
(n) Sedimentation techniques
(o) Specific surface
(p) Pore size
(q) void volume
(r) flow properties
(s) surface area
(t) arithmatic mean

(C) State true/false

1. The unit of particle size in micromeritics is most frequently used nanometer.
2. Ordinary microscope is suitable for determination of particle size in the range of 0.2 μm to 100 μm.
3. Microscopic method is used to determine the diameter of particle using only in two dimension (length and breath).
4. Sieves are generally used for grading coarse particles.
5. The particle size in the sub-sieve range may be determined by gravity sedimentation.
6. The sedimentation of particles whether the flow is turbulent or laminar is measured by the dimensionless Reynolds number.
7. Andreasen apparatus is used for determining particle volume.
8. Coulter counter is used for determining the particle volume.
9. Surface area of particles determined by sieving method.
10. Kozeny-Carman equation is derived from the Poiseuile equation is commonly used in air permeability methods for determination of partivcle size.
11. Bulk density is measured from the bulk volume and a weight of a dry powder in a graduated cylinder.
12. Free flowing powder are characterised by dustibility.
13. Flow properties of powder is improve using glidant.
14. The frictional forces in a loose powder measured in the form of compressibility index.
15. Specific bulk volume is proportional of bulk density is often called as bulkiness.
16. The volume of the spaces of powder is known as porosity.
17. The specific surface is the surface area per unit volume or per unit weight.

18. Reynolds number $(Re) = (vd\rho_0/\eta_0 0$

19. Stoke's equation $v = \dfrac{h}{t} = \dfrac{d_{st}^2 (\rho_s - \rho_o) g}{18 \eta_o}$

20. Poiseuille's equation $V = \dfrac{\pi d^4 \Delta P t}{128 \, l\eta}$

Answer (C) State true/false

1. F	2. T	3. T	4. T	5. T	6. T	7. F	8. T	9. F	10. T
11. T	12. T	13. T	14. F	15. F	16. T	17. T	18. T	19. T	20. T

❑❑❑

Table 1. Some commonly used physicochemical constants

Constant	Symbol	Value in C.G.S.	Value in S.I. units
Avogadro constant	N	6.02217×10^{23} mole^{-1}	6.022169×10^{23} mole^{-1}
Atomic mass unit	a.m.u.	1.666053×10^{-24} g	1.66053×10^{-27} Kg
Atmospheric pressure	P	1.01325×10^{6} dyne cm^{-2}	1.01325×10^{5} Nm^{-2}
Boltzmann constant	K	1.3800×10^{-16} erg K^{-1}	1.380×10^{-23} JK^{-1}
Charge on electron	e	4.80291×10^{-10} e.s.u.	1.60210×10^{-19} C
Faraday constant	F	$2.89461 \times 10^{+14}$ e.s.u.	9.6487×10^{7} C/kg equi.
Gas constant	R	8.3140×10^{7} ergK^{-1}mole^{-1}	8.3140 JK^{-1}mole^{-1}
Ice point	m.pt.	273.150 K	273.150 K
Mass of electran	m_e	9.10957×10^{-28} g	9.109557×10^{-31} kg
Mass of proton	m_p	1.67261×10^{-24} g	1.67261×10^{-27} kg
Mass of neutron	m_n	1.67492×10^{-24} g	1.67492×10^{-27}
Molar volume at STP	v	24414 cm^3	0.0224 m^3
Plank's constant	h	6.6261×10^{-27} erg sec.	6.6230×10^{-54} J sec
Rydberg constant	Rh	1.09737×10^{5} cm^{-1}	1.097373×107 m^{-1}
Speed of light	C	2.99790×10^{10} cm sec^{-1}	2.9979×10^{8} m sec^{-1}
Triple point of water	-	273.16 K	273.16 K

Table 2. Symbols and Abbreviation

Symbol	Abbreviations	Symbol	Abbreviations
At. Wt.	Atomic weight	Kcal	Killo calorie
Cm^3	Cubic centimeter	kJ	Killo joule
Cal.	Calorie	mg	Milli gram
DP	Discharge potential	M	Molar
$\propto$	Degree of Dissociation	m	Molal
Eq.	Equivalent	ml	Milli liter
Eq.wt.	Equivalent weight	Meq.	Milli equivalent
E.A.	Electron affinity	mM	Milli mole
g	Gram	N	Normal
IP	Ionisation potential	L	Litre
J	Joule	λ	Wavelength

Table 3. Greek alphabets

Greek name	Symbol	Greek name	Symbol
Alpha	α	Nu	ν
Beta	β	Xi	ξ
Gamma	γ	Omicron	O
Delta	Δ or δ	Pi	π
Epsilon	ε	Rho	ρ
Zeta	ζ	Sigma	Σ or σ
Eta	η	Tau	τ
Theta	θ	Upsilon	$\ni$
Iota	ι	Phi	ϕ
Kappa	κ	Chi	χ
Lambda	λ	Psi	ψ
Mu	μ	Omega	ω

Table 4. Physical quantities

Physical Quantities	Units	Symbol of units
Area	Square meter	m^2
Accelaration	Meter per second square	ms^{-2}
Amount	Mole	mole
Conductance	Siemens	$S(\Pi^{-2})$
Density	Kilogram per cubic	$kg\ m^{-3}$
Energy	Joule	$j(kgm^2s^{-2})$
Electric charge	Coulomb	coulomb
Electric potential	Volt	volt $(Kg\ ms^{-2})$
Force	Newton	$N\ (Kg\ m^2s^{-3}$
Frequency	Hertz	$Hz\ (s^{-1})$
Power	Watt	$W\ (Kg\ m^2s^{-3})$
Pressure	Pascal	$Pa\ (Nm^{-2})$
Resistance	Ohm	$Kg\ m^2s^{-3}A^{-2}$
Volume	Cubic meter	m^3
Velosity	Meter per second	

Table 5. Atomic number and atomic mass of elements.

Atomic number	Element	Symbol	Atomic weight
1	Hydrogen	H	1.0079
2	Helium	He	4.0026
3	Lithium	Li	6.9410
4	Beryllium	Be	9.0122
5	Boron	B	10.8110
6	Carbon	C	12.0011
7	Nitrogen	N	14.0070
8	Oxygen	O	15.9990
9	Fluorine	F	18.9980
10	Neon	Ne	20.1790
11	Sodium	Na	22.9900
12	Magnesium	Mg	24.3050
13	Aluminium	Al	26.9820
14	Silicone	Si	28.0860
15	Phosphorous	P	30.9740
16	Sulphur	S	32.0660
17	Chlorine	Cl	35.4530
18	Argon	Ar	39.9480
19	Potassium	K	39.0980

20	Calcium	Ca	40.0780
21	Scandium	Sc	44.9560
22	Titanium	Ti	47.8800
23	Vanadium	V	50.9420
24	Chromium	Cr	51.9960
25	Manganese	Mn	54.9380
26	Iron	Ir	55.8470
27	Cobalt	Co	58.9330
28	Nickel	Ni	58.6900
29	Copper	Cu	63.5460
30	Zinc	Zn	65.3900
31	Gallium	Ga	69.7230
32	Germanium	Ge	72.6100
33	Arsenic	As	74.9220
34	Selenium	Se	78.9600
35	Bromine	Br	79.9040
36	Krypton	Kr	83.8000
37	Rubidium	Rb	85.4680
38	Strontium	Sr	87.6200
39	Yttrium	Y	88.9060
40	Zirconium	Zr	91.2240
41	Niobium	Nb	92.9060
42	Molybdenum	Mo	95.9400
43	Technetium	Tc	98.9060
44	Ruthenium	Ru	101.0700
45	Rhodium	Rh	102.9100
46	Palladium	Pd	106.4200
47	Silver	Ag	107.8700
48	Cadmium	Cd	112.4100
49	Indium	In	114.8200
50	Tin	Sn	118.7100
51	Antimony	Sb	121.7500
52	Tellurium	Te	127.6000
53	Iodine	I	126.9000
54	Xenon	Xe	131.2900
55	Cesium	Cs	132.9100
56	Barium	Ba	137.3300
57	Lanthanum	La	138.9100
58	Cerium	Ce	140.1200
59	Praseodymium	Pr	140.9100
60	Neodymium	Nd	144.2400
61	Promethium	Pm	146.9200

62	Samarium	Sm	150.3600
63	Europium	Eu	151.9700
64	Gadolinium	Gd	157.2500
65	Terbium	Tb	158.9300
66	Dysprosium	Dy	162.5000
67	Holmium	Ho	164.9300
68	Erbium	Er	167.2600
69	Thulium	Tm	168.9300
70	Ytterbium	Yb	173.0400
71	Lutetium	Lu	174.9700
72	Hafnium	Hf	178.4900
73	Tantalum	Ta	180.9500
74	Tungsten	W	183.8500
75	Rhenium	Re	186.2000
76	Osmium	Os	190.2000
77	Iridium	Ir	192.2200
78	Platinum	Pt	195.0800
79	Gold	Au	196.9700
80	Mercury	Hg	200.5900
81	Thallium	Tl	204.3800
82	Lead	Pb	207.2000
83	Bismuth	Bi	208.9800
84	Polonium	Po	208.9800
85	Astatine	At	209.9900
86	Radon	Rn	222.0200
87	Francium	Fr	223.0200
88	Radium	Ra	226.0300
89	Actinium	Ac	227.0300
90	Thorium	Th	232.0400
91	Protactinium	Pa	231.0400
92	Uranium	U	238.0300
93	Neptunium	Np	237.0500
94	Plutonium	Pu	244.0600
95	Americium	Am	243.0600
96	Curium	Cm	247.0700
97	Berkelium	Bk	247.0700
98	Californium	Cf	251.0800
99	Einsteinium	Es	252.0800
100	Fermium	Fm	257.1000
101	Mendelevium	Md	258.1000
102	Nobelium	No	259.1000
103	Lawrencium	Lr	260.1000

104	Rutherfordium	Rf	261.1100
105	Hamium	Ha	262.1140
106	Unnilhexium	Unh	263.1180
107	Neilsbohrium	Ns	262.1200
108	Hassium	Hs	265.0000
109	Meitnerium	Mt	266.0000
110	Ununnilium	Uun	272.0000

Table 6. Surface tension of liquids at 20°C

Substance	Surface tension (dynes / cm.)	Substance	Surface tension (dynes / cm.)
Acetic acid	27.60	Formic acid	18.50
Acetone	23.71	Glycerin	63.40
Benzene	28.88	Heptane	19.0
Carbon tetrachloride	26.80	n-Hexane	22.60
Chlorobenzene	33.20	Methyl alcohol	28.40
Chloroform	27.10	Octane	21.80
Cyclohexane	25.30	n- Octane	26.50
Decane	23.90	Oleic acid	32.50
Dodecane	25.40	Perfluoroheptane	11.00
Ethyl acetate	25.90	Toluene	37.60
Ethyl alcohol	23.30	Water	72.80

Table 7. Interfacial tension of liquids against water at 20°C

Substance	Surface tension (dynes / cm.)	Substance	Surface tension (dynes / cm.)
Benzene	35.00	n-Hexane	50.80
Carbon tetrachloride	45.00	Murcury	428
Chloroform	32.80	n-Octanol	8.50
Decane	52.30	Oleic acid	15.6
Ether	10.70		

Table 8. Physical constant of water at different temperature

Temp. (°C)	Desity (g / ml)	Viscosity (cp)	Surface tension (dynes / cm.)	Vapor pressure (mmHg)	Refractive index
0	0.99987	1.7921	76.60	4.579	-
5	0.99999	1.5188	74.90	6.543	-
10	0.99973	1.3077	74.22	9.209	-
15	0.99913	1.1404	73.49	12.788	-
18	0.99862	1.0559	73.05	15.477	-
20	0.99823	1.0050	72.80	17.535	1.33300
21	0.99802	0.9810	-	18.650	1.33292
22	0.99780	0.9579	-	19.827	1.33283
23	0.99756	0.9358	-	21.068	1.33274
24	0.99732	0.9142	-	22.377	1.33264
25	0.99707	0.8937	71.97	23.756	1.33254
26	0.99681	0.8737	-	25.209	1.33243
27	0.99654	0.8545	-	26.739	1.33231
28	0.99626	0.8360	-	28.349	1.33219
29	0.99597	0.8180	-	30.043	1.33206
30	0.99567	0.8007	71.18	31.824	1.33192
31	0.99537	0.7840	-	33.695	-
32	0.99505	0.7679	-	35.663	1.33164
33	0.99473	0.7523	-	37.729	-
34	0.99440	0.7371	-	39.898	1.33136
35	0.99406	0.7225	-	42.175	-
37	0.99336	0.6947		47.067	-
39	0.99262	0.6685	-	52.442	-
40	0.99224	0.6560	69.56	55.324	1.33060
45	0.99025	0.5988	-	71.880	-
50	-	0.5494	67.91	-	-
60	-	0.4688	66.18	-	-
70	-	0.4062	64.40	-	-
80	-	0.3565	62.60	-	-
90	-	0.3165	-	-	-
100	-	0.2838	58.90	-	-

Table 9. Approximate viscosity of liquids.

Substance	Viscosity at °C				
	15	20	25	30	40
Acetic acid	-	-	1.555	1.040	-
Acetone	0.337	-	0.316	0.295	-
Benzene	-	0.652	-	0.503	0.503
n-Butyl alcohol	-	2.948	-	2.305	1.782
Carbon tetrachloride	-	0.969	-	0.843	0.739
Chlorobenzene	-	0.719	-	-	0.631
Chloroform	-	0.585	0.542	0.514	-
Ethyl acetate	-	0.455	0.441	0.412	-
Ethyl alcohol	-	1.202	-	1.004	0.834
Formic acid	-	1.805	-	1.465	1.209
Glycerin	-	1.495	0.948	0.629	-
Heptane	-	0.409	0.386	-	0.341
n-Hexane	-	0.325	0.295	-	-
Methyl alcohol	-	0.597	0.546	0.512	0.456
Propyl alcohol	2.860	-	-	1.772	-
Toluene	-	0.590	-	0.526	0.471
Turpentine	-	1.487	-	1.272	1.070